LIFE'S WORTH

A Critical Issues in Bioethics Series Book from

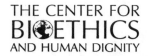

THE CENTER FOR
BIOETHICS
AND HUMAN DIGNITY

This volume continues the Center's second series of bioethics books. Whereas every book in the Center's well-established Horizons in Bioethics Series brings together an array of insightful writers to address important bioethical issues from a forward-looking Christian perspective, volumes in the Critical Issues in Bioethics Series have a different purpose. Each of these volumes features one or two authors bringing Christian perspectives into dialogue with other perspectives that are particularly influential today. The first volume addresses the field of bioethics broadly, while subsequent books focus on particular topics such as end-of-life issues.

Both series are projects of The Center for Bioethics and Human Dignity, an international center located just north of Chicago, Illinois, in the United States of America. The Center endeavors to bring Christian perspectives to bear on today's many pressing bioethical challenges. It pursues this task by developing two book series, nine audio series, nine video series, numerous conferences in different parts of the world, and a variety of other printed and computer-based resources. Through its membership/support program, the Center networks and provides resources for people interested in bioethical matters all over the world. Members/supporters receive the Center's international journal, *Ethics and Medicine,* the Center's newsletter, *Dignity,* special Center communications, an Internet News Service, and discounts on all Center resources and events.

For more information on membership in the Center or its various resources, including present or future books in the Critical Issues in Bioethics Series, contact the Center at:

The Center for Bioethics and Human Dignity
2065 Half Day Road
Bannockburn, IL 60015 USA
Phone: (847) 317-8180
Fax: (847) 317-8101
E-mail: cbhd@cbhd.org

Information and ordering is also available through the Center's World Wide Web site on the Internet: www.cbhd.org

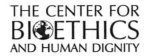

THE CENTER FOR
BIOETHICS
AND HUMAN DIGNITY

LIFE'S WORTH

The Case against Assisted Suicide

ARTHUR J. DYCK

WILLIAM B. EERDMANS PUBLISHING COMPANY
GRAND RAPIDS, MICHIGAN / CAMBRIDGE, U.K.

First published 2002 by Wm. B. Eerdmans Publishing Co.
2140 Oak Industrial Drive N.E., Grand Rapids, Michigan 49505 /
P.O. Box 163, Cambridge CB3 9PU U.K.

Printed in the United States of America

07 06 05 04 03 02   7 6 5 4 3 2 1

Library of Congress Cataloging-in-Publication Data

Dyck, Arthur J., 1932-
Life's worth: the case against assisted suicide / Arthur J. Dyck.
p.   cm.   (A Critical issues in bioethics series book)
Includes bibliographical references.
ISBN-10: 0-8028-4594-0 / ISBN-13: 978-0-8028-4594-8 (pbk.: alk. paper)
1. Assisted suicide — Moral and ethical aspects.
2. Assisted suicide — Religious aspects — Christianity.
3. Christian ethics.   I. Title.   II. Critical issues in bioethics series

R726.D937   2002
179.7 — dc21

2002029662

www.eerdmans.com

Dedicated to the memory of
Paul Ramsey
and
Joseph Stanton

Contents

Series Editors' Foreword

We live in an age when scientific knowledge has provided human beings with an unprecedented ability to manipulate life and death. In the West there has been a cultural shift from a so-called Judeo-Christian consensus to fragmented secular assumptions about the nature of human life, community, and "reproduction" as well as the practice of medicine and scientific research. There is little doubt that these changes in science and culture have fueled the controversies surrounding abortion, physician-assisted suicide, genetic engineering, the patient-doctor relationship, reproductive technologies, cloning, and the allocation of health care resources, to name just a few.

Bioethics is the interdisciplinary study of these and other issues of life and health. It involves an attempt to discover normative guidelines built on sound moral foundations.

The purpose of this series is to bring thoughtful and biblically informed Christian voices in bioethics into dialogue with other voices that are influential today. As Christians we believe that human persons are made in the image of God and for that reason their lives are sacred. We also believe that God's entire creation was made for a purpose, and we discover this purpose from the Holy Scripture as well as philosophical reflections on the nature of things. Because we live in a pluralist society, we believe that it is our responsibility to explain why all people should take Christian perspectives into account. Such is the case not least because these perspectives have shaped so much of Western culture, especially its assumptions about human dignity. Accordingly, the books in this series will be useful to those who do not share our theological commitments. They can be read side by side with books espousing secular or other perspectives and are ideal for bioethics courses in nontheological as well as theological settings.

Because bioethics is theoretical as well as practical, the authors in this series are committed to providing a principled case for their perspectives as well as suggestions and insights on how scientists and/or health care practitioners may employ these principles in a laboratory and/or clinical setting. In addition, we believe that pastors, students, professors, and others will profit from these books. C. S. Lewis warned of a future in which "Man's final conquest has proved to be the abolition of Man." The purpose of this series is to help forestall or even prevent such a future.

DENNIS HOLLINGER
Vice Provost
Professor of Christian Ethics
Messiah College

FRANCIS J. BECKWITH
James Madison Fellow in
    Constitutional Studies &
    Political Thought
Princeton University

Introduction

"Favoring physician-assisted suicide [hereafter PAS] is intuitive, self-evident; it is a matter of compassion." That is what one of my students recently claimed, and his view is shared by others. "After all," he went on to argue, "what else would any humane person do but assist those who are suffering and terminally ill to die if they wish such assistance?"

Such a view is certainly understandable. Consider the situation of Sidney Cohen who was told by his physician that he had cancer and that he would die a painful death in less than three months. The cancer was diagnosed in November and by January 1 Sidney Cohen described himself as "bed bound by pain and weakness, having been able to drink only water for six weeks . . . desperate, isolated and frightened" and wishing for euthanasia.[1] If this is what one knows about Sidney Cohen's condition and his feelings about it, does it not seem inhumane to deny him a painless death and, if the prognosis is correct, spare him the suffering he is slated to endure for another month?

But that is not the whole story. What we have before us is a static snapshot of this man. Indeed, this description is only part of what Sidney Cohen wrote about himself *eight* months after he was diagnosed with cancer and given three months to live. On January 1, he tells us, "I truly wished that euthanasia could have been administered."[2] But it wasn't! So what has transpired in the months following January 1? In Sidney Cohen's own words,

---

1. Robert G. Twycross, "Where There Is Hope, There Is Life: A View from the Hospice," in John Keown, ed., *Euthanasia Examined: Ethical, Clinical and Legal Perspectives* (Cambridge: Cambridge University Press, 1995), p. 142.

2. Twycross, "Where There Is Hope," p. 142.

I now know that only death is inevitable and since coming under the care of the MacMillan Service [hospice homecare] my pain has been relieved completely, my ability to enjoy life restored and my fears of an agonizing end allayed. . . . I'm still alive today. My weight and strength have increased since treatment made it possible to eat normally and I feel that I'm living a full life, worth living. My wife and I have come to accept that I'm dying and we can now discuss it openly between ourselves and with the staff of the MacMillan Service, which does much to ease our anxieties.

My experiences have served to convince me that euthanasia, even if voluntary, is fundamentally wrong and I'm now staunchly against it on religious, moral, intellectual and spiritual grounds. My wife's views have changed similarly.[3]

Clearly there are those who, hearing a description of someone in Sidney Cohen's condition on that January 1, are convinced that honoring his request to assist him to die then, rather than suffer longer, is the morally appropriate, compassionate response. Indeed, one hears the argument accompanying such case descriptions that it is reasonable that no one would want to live under those circumstances. At the same time, the opponents of PAS and euthanasia can provide snapshots of cases helped by hospice homecare or other medical interventions, documenting peaceful deaths and/or gratitude for dying relatively free of anxiety, and virtually or completely free of pain.

But such snapshots, or even fuller case descriptions, do not settle the issues raised by the experiences of Sidney Cohen and others diagnosed as terminally ill or suffering from severely debilitating illnesses. What should such individuals ask of their caregivers and loved ones, and what kind of care ought to be offered? How should such seriously ill individuals relate to others, and how should others relate to them? What moral responsibilities do caregivers and those being cared for have to one another and to their communities? What moral responsibilities do communities have toward the severely ill and those who provide care for them?

Some in effect argue that these questions are not relevant for those who are dying unless they want to put these questions to themselves. As a dying person, they say, "I will and I should act on the basis of my own snapshot of myself, and on my own view of whether my life should continue beyond a certain time. And, furthermore, I should have the right to receive assistance to discontinue life if and when I request it. So why even write a book trying to persuade me to think ever so carefully about whether or not PAS is ever morally justifiable and whether PAS should or should not be against the law? I

3. Twycross, "Where There Is Hope," pp. 142-43.

2

should not have the manner of my dying dictated by governments and by legislation, once I am in a condition in which it is rational for me to seek to end my life, or to seek assistance to accomplish that quickly and painlessly."

But a decision to request PAS is influenced and shaped by assessments that are not simply those of the patient making the request. What patients regard as reasonable is not solely based on their own thinking, their own feeling, or their independent assessment of their illness and its future course. To regard oneself as terminally ill is, certainly to begin with, usually and largely based on a medical assessment, a diagnosis by a physician or physicians. To conclude that any given symptom, such as extreme pain, will persist until death, is largely a function of a prognosis and can be largely, if not entirely, a function of the quality of care and knowledge of the caregivers. A change in care, as in Sidney Cohen's case, can change one's condition, one's self-assessment, and even what one considers to be reasonable care for those who are dying. Furthermore, what is perceived as reasonable may be unreasonable because the diagnoses and/or prognoses that shape one's perceptions are mistaken. Consider the case of Mr. CJ:

> Mr. CJ, aged 48, was diagnosed as having cancer of the right maxillary antrum in October 1989. He was given two months to live and told that he would go blind. Thirteen months later he had not gone blind and had improved sufficiently to return to work.[4]

In the Netherlands and the American state of Oregon, given this man's diagnosis and prognosis, he is clearly eligible, provided he is not diagnosed as being depressed, to receive medical assistance to end his life were he to request such assistance. In Oregon, he is not legally required to consult with his family or friends. Without knowing that he would not actually go blind, would not die in two months, and would not lose but gain the strength to resume his occupation, there are those who regard any desire of his to have his life end as undoubtedly rational, and helping him as compassionate.

I cite this case to encourage a careful reading of the issues at stake for individuals and communities. And so I am asking my reader, if you were CJ, would you have preferred to have a ban on PAS so you could predictably return to your work, or no ban so that you could accept the risks of error and gain the freedom to cope as you would choose? You might, after all, be the kind of individual who would pursue second and third opinions and these might detect the error, or buy you the time to feel your strength returning while suffering no loss of sight. I want you to think also about those who

4. Twycross, "Where There Is Hope," p. 158.

3

would prefer returning to work to ending their lives, but yet would choose assisted suicide because of the terror about going blind, and because, for whatever reason, they do not discover that this prognosis is mistaken. In short, moral disapproval of PAS and laws against it on the whole increase individual choices even for individuals who oppose such laws.

The reasons for this are not limited to the inevitability of incorrect diagnoses and prognoses. What happens to individuals and what choices they make will be quite different, depending upon what laws are in place, and what choices are encouraged by physicians, whether explicitly or implicitly. Compare, for example, a sample population of AIDS patients in the United Kingdom with AIDS patients in the Netherlands. A study of 110 patients cared for in three different AIDS treatment centers in London found that, though suicide and euthanasia are discussed with all patients as a matter of policy, only 10 percent of patients addressed this "in significant terms," and only two of the 110 patients "pursued euthanasia as a realistic option."[5] One of them never took up the offer to contact the Voluntary Euthanasia Society, and dropped the whole idea of euthanasia after admission to a hospice. The other instance of wishing to pursue euthanasia had only been initiated at the time the study was reported, and so there was no outcome to report at that time. Given that the palliative care for these 110 patients is good, the author of this study, R. George, concludes that, "In the last month of life, euthanasia is a serious option in only a small minority, and in our experience this is symptomatic of an unresolved agenda, rather than a considered and clear choice."[6] These findings contrast sharply with what happens in the Netherlands. There 30 percent of AIDS patients receive euthanasia, presumably upon request if it is done in accord with legally accepted guidelines.[7]

From these data, we can see that individual choices are influenced and shaped by the type of care provided and accepted, legally as well as morally, by physicians and the larger society. In the Netherlands, only about 25 percent of its doctors have received training in cancer pain management.[8] This lack of knowledge is reflected in patient care: a survey of a large teaching hospital in Amsterdam revealed that only about 25 percent of cancer patients received "optimal treatment for their pain, and that over half of them were treated inappropriately. . . . Forty percent of doctors were unaware of the pain (some-

5. Twycross, "Where There Is Hope," p. 152, citing R. George, "Euthanasia: The AIDS Dimension," in N. M. de S. Cameron, ed., *Death without Dignity* (Edinburgh: Rutherford House Books, 1990), pp. 176-95.
6. Twycross, "Where There Is Hope," p. 152.
7. Twycross, "Where There Is Hope," p. 153.
8. Twycross, "Where There Is Hope," p. 159.

times severe) which their cancer patients were experiencing."[9] Whatever their convictions about PAS and euthanasia, individuals simply will be much more likely to consider these as options and much more likely to choose them in the Netherlands than in the situations encountered by those patients in London. It is not realistic to describe these choices as completely "private" or "self-determined." These choices will vary as human relations, medical knowledge, and what is lawful varies. Accordingly, the choice to favor or to oppose PAS and laws that permit it is a choice as to the kind of community one will inhabit, and the way in which physicians and others will relate to one another and to those who are severely ill or regarded as dying. That same study in London found that 50 percent of the patients experienced significant changes in their "attitude and world view in the last three months of life," moving toward an acceptance of their death and "psychological and spiritual peace." As the author of the study notes, "The introduction of voluntary euthanasia [would] mean that many people will be denying themselves this crucial time when half of them are likely to have major shifts in their emotional and spiritual attitudes."[10]

But even those who find these experiences in the last three months of life very desirable, even praiseworthy, may not be moved to prefer a community that legally forbids PAS and hence also euthanasia. Some, whose views we will be discussing later in this work, still would prefer the freedom to decide whether they will live out their last months, and whether they will need the assistance of a physician to die quickly and painlessly when that seems best to them, given their particular ailment and their own perceptions of its effects. Six rather well-known American philosophers expressed this view in a brief to the United States Supreme Court: "Each individual has a right to make the 'most intimate and personal choices central to personal dignity and autonomy.' That right encompasses the right to exercise some control over the time and manner of one's death."[11] These philosophers asked the United States Supreme Court to join the Ninth and Second Circuit Courts of Appeals in declaring any flat legal prohibition of PAS to be unconstitutional.[12] Arguments

9. Twycross, "Where There Is Hope," p. 159.

10. Twycross, "Where There Is Hope," p. 153, citing R. George, "Euthanasia: The AIDS Dimension."

11. "Brief of Ronald Dworkin, Thomas Nagel, Robert Nozick, John Rawls, Thomas Scanlon, and Judith Jarvis Thomson as Amicus Curiae, in Support of Respondents," *Issues in Law and Medicine* 15, no. 2 (Fall 1999): 196.

12. The U.S. Supreme Court did not accept the reasoning of the six philosophers named in footnote 11 above, overturning the Ninth Circuit Court in *Washington v. Glucksberg,* 117 S.Ct. 2258 (1997) and overturning the Second Circuit Court in *Vacco v. Quill,* 117

for such a prohibition would, in the view of these philosophers, necessarily be based on contested religious or ethical convictions that any given terminally ill patient may not share or accept. The absolute ban of PAS would then be taking sides in what should be regarded as a very private and personal matter that should remain free, in some circumstances, from government interference. The Supreme Court rejected that argument.[13] The idea that killing someone under mutually agreed upon circumstances could be socially and legally tolerated is not new. In the United States, duels were common from the time of the first settlement: a duel occurred in Plymouth in 1621.[14] This kind of combat for the sake of defending one's honor or dignity developed from earlier, medieval forms of judicial combat to decide controversies such as guilt for crimes and ownership of disputed lands. They were frequent in the United States during the eighteenth and early nineteenth centuries and usually lethal. In the most notorious case, Alexander Hamilton was killed by Aaron Burr in 1804 at the same place his eldest son had died in a duel three years earlier. The District of Columbia outlawed dueling in 1839, and since the American Civil War, all the states have passed laws penalizing duels.

But why speak of dueling? One could argue that there is no reason to ban it since it was voluntary and only the participants risked or suffered death. Yet it came to be socially disapproved and banned throughout the world. The claim that this practice should be allowed to preserve one's dignity as an individual did not prevail. Indeed, in France, dueling was so popular that Henry IV made it punishable by death. Why? Too many people were being killed. And, in the nineteenth and twentieth centuries there were notable organizations dedicated to fostering disapproval of dueling. That is not surprising. For the question as to when killing and being killed are to be practiced and condoned is an abiding question for communities as a whole, as well as for their individual members.

The fact then, that PAS as a practice evokes differences of opinion and belief should not automatically lead one to accept a proposal that, on the surface, would appear to harm no one. I refer to the suggestion that only those who wish PAS would have legal permission; others are free to shun the practice. As this book should make evident, such a legal and moral structure is as much a choice about the kind of community all of its members will experience as a choice for a legal and moral structure designed to ban assisted sui-

---

S.Ct. 2293 (1997). In these two decisions, the Supreme Court upheld the constitutionality of the laws banning assisted suicide in Washington and New York.

13. See *Glucksberg*, 2269-71.

14. See the entry "Duel" in *Funk & Wagnalls Standard Reference Encyclopedia*, vol. 8.

cide in all circumstances. Given the debate over PAS, nothing less than what kind of community should prevail is being contested.

The central argument of this book is that there is a solid moral and practical basis for the laws against assisted suicide that now exist in the United States and elsewhere. Furthermore, in the current debate that case is not being made in a convincing way. The members of any community need to know the reasons why everyone should want to prevent suicide and what laws are necessary to sustain such efforts and achieve a high degree of success. At the same time, all of us need to know whether the traditions that favor PAS will undermine not only efforts to curb suicide but also killing more generally. This is a real possibility since, as I argue, the moral and practical bases for the laws against assisted suicide are also the bases for the laws that specify and punish what constitutes murder.

It is not enough, however, to show that the reasons for laws preventing suicide are sufficiently similar to those justifying laws against murder, and hence should have the same high level of support from the general populace. There are now philosophers who claim that the reason that killing is wrong is that the one being killed does not wish to be killed. On this view, assisting individuals to die who are capable of assessing the value of their own lives, and who wish to die, is neither wrongful killing, nor wrongful assistance of those who kill themselves.[15] As I will suggest in more detail later, this way of thinking is quite different from the moral traditions that provide a rationale for our current legal protections of human life. Current laws presuppose a shared moral outlook that characterizes life as sacred, and as an inalienable human right. Killing a human being cannot presently be legally justified on the grounds that the individual who was killed wanted to die.[16] At stake then in the debate over assisted suicide is nothing less than a shift away from a moral

15. See, for example, Tom Beauchamp and James F. Childress, *Principles of Biomedical Ethics*, 4th ed. (New York: Oxford University Press, 1994); John Harris, "Euthanasia and the Value of Life," in John Keown, ed., *Euthanasia Examined: Ethical, Clinical and Legal Perspectives* (Cambridge: Cambridge University Press, 1995), pp. 6-22; Frances M. Kamm, "Physician-Assisted Suicide, Euthanasia, and Intending Death," in M. P. Battin, R. Rhodes, and S. Silvers, eds., *Physician-Assisted Suicide: Expanding the Debate* (New York: Routledge, 1998), pp. 28-62. The reader should note that the 5th edition of Beauchamp and Childress was issued too late in 2001 to be included in this book. However, I have read the relevant sections, and there is no change in this argument.

16. Jack Kevorkian could not successfully defend his act of euthanasia by appealing to the desire of the individual who was killed by lethal injection: He is serving a term in prison for murder. That the law against homicide does not accept as a defense against murder the fact that the one killed desired to be killed is clearly emphasized by the Supreme Court decision in *Glucksberg*.

structure that is at once the expression of our shared humanity and also the source of the responsibilities and rights necessary to sustain individual and communal life. Or to put the issue differently: Does the kind of thinking that permits assisted suicide provide a moral basis for protecting the preciousness of human life or does it fail to provide a moral structure that will predictably protect individual and communal life? What I will argue is that there is a moral structure we share as human beings. We pay homage to this shared moral structure when we praise individuals for being humane and condemn action deemed to be inhumane. Some crimes are so inhumane that we characterize them as crimes against humanity. This same moral structure, for reasons I will later suggest, is the basis for laws against homicide and does not support the legalization of assisted suicide. The rationale for assisted suicide sets aside this moral structure, substituting an account of moral agency that will not, in my view, predictably sustain individual and communal life, nor the laws against homicide and euthanasia.

The argument of this book will proceed in four stages. Human suffering is what launches any consideration of assisted suicide. It is the suffering of the terminally ill that is the main focus of those who suggest that PAS be declared a constitutional right, or at least be legally permitted. To begin with then, it is important to examine the reasons that some physicians, moral philosophers, and theologians are urging that assisted suicide be one of the services that physicians offer those patients who are deemed to be suffering and reasonably wishing to die. No less important are the reasons other physicians, philosophers, and theologians urge alternative ways to relieve the suffering of patients. These responses include: withholding or withdrawing of treatment regarded as far more burdensome than beneficial, or as burdensome only; the administration of pain relief to the extent necessary to relieve pain; and any care necessary to deal with other possible sources of suffering. I call these responses to the pain and suffering of patients who are terminally ill "comfort-only care."

But even if one grants that there are these alternatives to PAS, and that they can be quite effective, the debate does not cease, but moves on to another stage. If it is morally and legally acceptable to dispense with life-sustaining interventions in certain conditions, and to relieve pain even to the extent that life is sometimes shortened, why not also accept assisted suicide as quicker, surer, and hence a more merciful way to end suffering? There are, as I will indicate, strong, long-standing objections to equating comfort-only, sometimes life-shortening treatment, with interventions that intentionally end life with known, lethal means. Chapter Two indicates ways in which comfort-only treatment differs morally from PAS and euthanasia. The chapter ends with a challenge to the relevance of the differences I have specified.

8

Once again, the debate over PAS does not end but requires the consideration of further arguments, both of which are based upon autonomy. The first is an argument as to what makes killing wrong when it is wrong; the second is an argument to the effect that any ban of all assisted suicides, and all the arguments used to justify such a ban, impose on me a view of how I should die that I should be able to determine free from legal interference. How and when I should die is a personal matter of individual conscience. Those who reject PAS need not request it and so are free to die in accord with their most deeply held convictions. The response to this mode of thinking requires more than the usual criticisms of it. And so in this third chapter, I will depict more fully the moral structure underlying homicide law and the current laws against assisted suicide and euthanasia. This, I will suggest, is a moral structure that we share as human beings. Given this moral structure, banning assisted suicide and euthanasia are not unwelcome impositions, but part of a long-standing effort to protect freedom, as well as life.

This moral structure being depicted and defended in Chapter Three and embedded in current American law, draws on certain concepts and affirmations found in Christian theological and scriptural thought, and found as well in Western philosophy. But the claims being made in the *sources* of anyone's thinking are distinguished from *warrant* for one's claims, whatever their sources. The arguments in Chapter Three that serve as the warrant for the moral structure inherent in current homicide law are factual and logical. Indeed, I agree that this moral structure is essential to individual and communal life and is to be found wherever communities exist and persist.[17] Furthermore, the human rights supported by this moral structure are rights justly owed to us as human beings, whatever our loyalties to particular faiths, religious or nonreligious.

However, I do view the moral structure, and the warrant offered for it in Chapter Three, as compatible with long-standing and persistent ways of thinking within Christianity. To defend that view is one of the major purposes of the fourth and concluding chapter. In carrying out this purpose, the chapter gives an account of the major reasons found in Christian thought for supporting this moral structure and opposing PAS and euthanasia. This last chapter ends by pointing to certain Christian beliefs that provide comfort and hope to those who are suffering, dying, or experiencing the death of loved ones.

---

17. For a more complete account of these moral requisites of individual and communal life, see Arthur J. Dyck, *Rethinking Rights and Responsibilities: The Moral Bonds of Community* (Cleveland: Pilgrim Press, 1994). A revised edition is forthcoming from Georgetown University Press.

CHAPTER ONE

Responding to Suffering:
Physician-Assisted Suicide versus
Comfort-Only Care

Physicians have always viewed the alleviation of suffering, as well as attempts to cure, as obligatory.[1] In the Netherlands, this has come to include PAS and euthanasia. These practices were officially condoned by the Dutch Supreme Court in 1984 when it held that a doctor who kills a patient may invoke the defense of necessity to justify the killing, in certain circumstances, and thus satisfy the Dutch Penal Code then, but no longer, proscribing euthanasia.[2] In the United States, physicians have begun openly to advocate PAS. A committee of twelve physicians published a set of recommendations in 1989 to guide physicians in the care of what they called "hopelessly ill patients." Included among the kinds of care being suggested was PAS. Ten of the twelve physicians took the view "that it is not immoral for a physician to assist in the rational suicide of a terminally ill person."[3] These physicians made it abundantly clear that they were not equating PAS with their other recommendations to provide patients with maximal pain relief and

1. See, for example, Edmund D. Pellegrino, "Euthanasia and Assisted Suicide," in John F. Kilner, Arlene B. Miller, and Edmund D. Pellegrino, eds., *Dignity and Dying: A Christian Appraisal* (Grand Rapids: Eerdmans, 1996), pp. 105-19.

2. For an account of the legal situation and practices relative to PAS and euthanasia, see Henck Jochemsen, "The Netherlands Experiment," in Kilner et al., eds., *Dignity and Dying*, pp. 165-79; see also John Keown, "Euthanasia in the Netherlands: Sliding Down the Slippery Slope?" in John Keown, ed., *Euthanasia Examined: Ethical, Clinical and Legal Perspectives* (Cambridge: Cambridge University Press, 1995), pp. 261-96.

3. S. H. Wanzer et al., "The Physician's Responsibility Toward Hopelessly Ill Patients: A Second Look," *New England Journal of Medicine* 320 (1989): 844-49.

flexibly adjusted efforts to minimize suffering even if such actions aimed at comfort should shorten life.

In 1991 public advocacy for PAS as an extension of the services physicians should render suffering patients was greatly heightened when Timothy E. Quill, a medical doctor, published a case in which he assisted in the suicide of one of his patients.[4] Since this published case has been much cited, and since Quill presents a clear and plausible rationale for his actions, it makes sense to center this chapter around his rationale. Quill's case is also something of a paradigm case, containing many of the elements that lead some physicians and others to favor and advocate for PAS.

The Case of Diane: A Rationale for PAS

Quill's patient, Diane, was diagnosed as having acute myelomonocytic leukemia. The odds given her of surviving painful and prolonged treatment were 25 percent. Without treatment, she would have days or weeks, or, at most, a few months to live. With some reservations, Quill accepted her refusal of treatment in order to avoid the suffering she anticipated from a treatment she believed would fail.

But Diane's wishes did not stop there. Quill had made arrangements for hospice care, and had made, in his view, every effort to persuade her to remain there. Instead, she expressed the wish "to take her life" and do so "in the least painful way possible." Quill defends her wish as follows: "Knowing of her desire for independence and her decision to stay in control, I thought this request made perfect sense."[5] For Quill, taking one's life can be reasonable, but a physician is needed to confirm whether leaving comfort care is, given the circumstances, reasonable in each individual case. Quill does speak of his efforts in Diane's case to ensure, by having conversations, that her judgment was not colored by despair, and that all other alternatives had truly been found wanting. Quill sees himself as extending the services physicians should offer their patients. Those services should go beyond comfort care when care is no longer efficacious, or curative efforts are no longer accepted by the patient. In Quill's own words, "Diane taught me about the

4. Timothy Quill, "Death and Dignity: A Case of Individualized Decision Making," *New England Journal of Medicine* 324, no. 10 (March 7, 1991): 691-94. The publicity around Jack Kevorkian's practice of PAS and ultimately euthanasia seems to have encouraged opposition to PAS as well as advocacy, but it is difficult to judge without hard data. In the case of Quill a great deal of published advocacy and criticisms addressed Quill's action.

5. Quill, "Death and Dignity," p. 693.

range of help I can provide if I know people and if I allow them to say what they really want."[6]

Quill is explicit about indicating the kind of help his patient required once she had chosen suicide: (1) assuring that the suicide would be effective so that the lingering death feared by Diane would not occur; (2) avoiding a violent death with its adverse effects on the patient's family; (3) giving Diane the requisite information, in this instance calling attention to the Hemlock Society; (4) prescribing and indicating the dosages of barbiturates required to commit suicide as quickly and painlessly as possible; and (5) comforting her family. To help Diane and the family still further, Quill does not inform the medical examiner that a suicide has taken place, listing the cause of death as acute leukemia. By doing this, he protects Diane's family, as well as his own, from investigations and any possible criminal charges. Quill was clearly uncomfortable about the deceit he deemed necessary, given New York State's prohibition of assisted suicide. That was also evident later when he challenged New York's law, seeking to have PAS legalized. His challenge was upheld in 1996 by the Second Circuit Court of Appeals in the decision bearing his name, *Quill v. Vacco;* that decision was struck down by the Supreme Court in 1997.[7]

There are at least three significant reasons Quill has for engaging in PAS and for urging legal permission to do so: (1) accepting the wishes of patients who are suffering; (2) circumstances that make suicide a rational act; (3) going beyond the alleviation of suffering by eliminating or avoiding it altogether. These bear careful scrutiny, for they are prominent in the debates regarding PAS.

The Wishes of Patients

Quill is very clear that he has for a long time advocated active and informed choices by patients with regard to treatment or nontreatment. These choices by themselves need not be made with the intention of ending one's life. Patients may reject treatment they view as unduly burdensome or of little or no compensating benefit, everything considered. Quill notes, however, that he has also long advocated "a patient's right to die with as much control and dignity as possible."[8] If one is to actualize that right, as Quill understands it, the

---

6. Quill, "Death and Dignity," p. 694.

7. The Supreme Court struck down *Quill v. Vacco* 80 F. 3rd 716 (2nd Cir. 1996) in *Vacco v. Quill,* 117 S.Ct. 2293 (1997).

8. Quill, "Death and Dignity," p. 692.

choices open to patients must extend beyond the refusal of treatment to the employment of the means necessary and sufficient to bring about death when and how one wishes. For Quill, that encompasses the choice to request PAS. Indeed, in a later work detailing criteria that would justify PAS and legal permission for carrying it out in a given case, the free will, not advance directives, and the undistorted judgment of patients, head the list.[9]

Quill seems to take for granted that respecting the wishes of patients has the weight of a strict moral obligation. There certainly is a voluminous literature in bioethics that refers to this obligatory respect for the choices of patients as respect for autonomy. Indeed, autonomy has been widely depicted as a moral principle.[10] This is a problematic proposition to be analyzed in Chapter Three.

Bearing in mind that these wishes which Quill and others would have physicians honor are those of patients who are suffering and who have sought the assistance of physicians for some kind of relief, how should one respond to these wishes? Do such wishes provide a compelling reason for a physician's aid in ending one's life? Dame Cicely Saunders founded the contemporary hospice movement to relieve pain and suffering so effectively that patients would not only have an alternative to suicide and euthanasia, but would not even wish to end their lives in these ways. She can certainly provide us with dramatic success stories like the following one:

> A family doctor asked our clinic staff to visit one young woman in her forties whose pain and vomiting had become uncontrollable. We discovered later that by this time her distress was so great that not only had she attempted suicide but when she failed the family had discussed whether they should not add together all the pills and try to end her life. We were not told this until a year later. Instead she spent most of that year at home with her family, able once again to enjoy life, to work and even to shop and care for the three children. She overcame her fear of hospitals, attended our Out-Patients, came for one short stay to re-establish control of her vomiting and finally came in peacefully for her last two weeks. One of the things she said to us at [this] stage was, "The children are a year older." It was when she was dying that we were told of the despairing attempt of a year before. We asked if she had ever again demanded for her life to be ended. We were told, "Never. Not after the Sister came, because [I] never had any more pain." We

---

9. Timothy E. Quill, *Death and Dignity: Making Choices and Taking Charge* (New York: W. W. Norton, 1993), pp. 161-65.

10. See, for example, Tom Beauchamp and James F. Childress, *Principles of Biomedical Ethics,* 4th ed. (New York: Oxford University Press, 1994).

know that this family has really begun to live once more, as her husband calls frequently at a social club at the Hospice designed for such informal "follow-up." How different it would have been if they had remembered only the bewilderment and guilt that follow a suicide or the course they had discussed. And they all needed that extra year.[11]

In this case, we gain a perspective on the wishes of patients very different from the one exhibited by Quill. For one thing, wishes are portrayed as subject to change. A wish for suicide can become a wish to live longer. For another thing, the wishes of a given patient are dependent on the activities of others. This woman would not have lived had her family decided to assist her in taking a sufficiently lethal dose in accord with her wishes at the time. This woman might not have changed her wishes had no one attempted and succeeded to relieve her of the pain and vomiting that she had been suffering. When a physician like Quill relinquishes his advocacy for treatment in the first instance, and for comfort-only treatment in the second instance, there is no way of knowing how well and how long Diane might have lived.

Quill would no doubt object to any suggestion that Diane would have changed her mind about what she wanted. After all, she is not the same person being discussed by Saunders, and Quill had, in his view, made a good-faith effort to have her accept treatment, and when that failed, to accept hospice care, an effort that also failed. There is no way of knowing whether Saunders could have prevented Diane from committing suicide, on her own or with the aid of another physician. What we do know, however, is that Quill did not do all that he could or should have done to actualize his claim that he had left the door open for Diane to change her mind about committing suicide. In fact, his responses to Diane can be viewed as influencing the persistence of her wish to commit suicide.

In an analysis of the case of Diane as described by Quill, Dr. Patricia Wesley, a psychiatrist, points out:

> It is frighteningly naïve to assume that when our guide to medical practice is "doing what the patient wants," we will escape the imposition of the physician's values on the clinical encounter. Personal values can be sequestered in the question not asked, or the gentle challenge not posed, when both should have been.[12]

11. Cicely M. S. Saunders, "The Care of the Dying Patient and His Family," in S. J. Reiser, W. J. Curran, and A. J. Dyck, eds., *Ethics in Medicine: Historical Perspectives and Contemporary Concerns* (Cambridge, Mass.: MIT Press, 1977), p. 513.

12. Patricia Wesley, "Dying Safely," *Issues in Law and Medicine* 8, no. 3 (1993): 467.

Quill believes that the request to be aided in taking Diane's life made "perfect sense," and he responds to the request by referring her to the Hemlock Society and describing what he did as "helpful." In Wesley's view, these responses conveyed the message, albeit implicitly, perhaps unwittingly, that Quill agreed that "if you cannot be fully independent, you are better off dead."[13] Wesley adds:

> In making this referral and describing it as "helpful," Dr. Quill once again powerfully shaped the clinical interaction between himself and his patient. It is not a neutral act to refer a patient contemplating suicide to the Hemlock Society. . . . It renders incoherent to us, as possibly it did to Diane, Dr. Quill's claim that he had left the door open for her to change her mind.[14]

Wesley wonders whether the result would have been different if Quill had recommended a support group of cancer patients instead. We know from the study cited in the Introduction that the total context will influence what patients wish and what happens to these wishes in the course of interaction with physicians. I refer to the research revealing that 30 percent of AIDS patients in the Netherlands have their lives ended; in a hospice in London only 10 percent of their AIDS patients seriously addressed the possibility of ending their lives, and only one patient out of 110 in the study had not clearly dropped the idea at the time these results were published.[15]

Another psychiatrist, Dr. Herbert Hendin, thinks that neither Quill nor Diane came to grips with the fear of death. He notes that

> many patients and physicians displace anxieties about death onto the circumstances of dying — pain, dependence, loss of dignity, as well as the unpleasant side effects resulting from medical treatment, or, for the physician, frustration at not being able to offer a sure cure. Focusing on or becoming enraged at the process distracts from the fear of death itself.[16]

Hendin elaborates on this point by describing how he assists patients to confront such fears and shifts the focus of the patient on what can be achieved with what life still may have to offer. The case of Diane interests him so much because he had a patient, Tim, who had the same type of cancer with the

13. Patricia Wesley, "Dying Safely," p. 483.

14. Patricia Wesley, "Dying Safely," p. 483.

15. R. George, "Euthanasia: The AIDS Dimension," in N. M. de S. Cameron, ed., *Death without Dignity* (Edinburgh: Rutherford House Books, 1990), pp. 176-95.

16. Herbert Hendin, "Seduced by Death: Doctors, Patients and the Dutch Cure," *Issues in Law and Medicine* 10, no. 2 (1994): 128.

same 25 percent chance of survival. Tim's first reaction to this prospect was a fixation on committing suicide and a wish for support in accomplishing it. In Hendin's own words,

> At first he [Tim] could not consider how he felt about death and its meaning to him but remained preoccupied with concerns about being dependent and unwilling to tolerate the symptoms of his disease or the side effects of proposed treatment. Once we could talk about the possibility or likelihood of his dying — what it meant to him in terms of separation and bodily disintegration — his desperate avoidance subsided. He decided to undergo medical treatment, complained relatively little about the unpleasant side effects, and used the remaining months of his life to connect with his wife and parents in ways that were moving and meaningful to him. Two days before he died, Tim talked of what he would have missed without the opportunity for a loving parting.[17]

Hendin does not regard the fears surrounding what to expect from the dying process as unreasonable, but the fear of death itself amplified them. Treatment is more bearable when freed from the fear of imminent death.

We can see that Hendin approaches a situation like that of Diane's much differently than Quill did. One cannot conclusively argue that Hendin could have successfully changed Diane's wishes. What does appear to be highly likely, however, is that Tim's desire for suicide was very likely to persist in the absence of Hendin's efforts. In any event, the wishes of patients, like their pain and suffering, are very much dependent on the relationships they have with their physicians and other individuals at the time they are faced with the prospect of dying. No simple appeal to the wishes of patients can by itself justify assent by a physician or anyone else, to their requests for assistance in committing suicide.

At this point in the discussion, Quill could say that he does not base a decision to assist in ending a patient's life simply on their express wishes. As in the case of Diane, Quill would insist that such a decision must rest as well on the reasonableness of the request.

The Rationality of Suicide

As previously noted, Quill explicitly regards Diane's choice of suicide as "making perfect sense." He expresses this belief by assuring us that he knew

17. Hendin, "Seduced by Death," p. 128

how much she desired independence and control over her situation. Physicians should, of course, make certain that the judgment of a patient is not driven by despair — he does not mention fear of death — and that all other alternatives have been "found wanting." Among the additional criteria for PAS advocated by Quill is that the patient's condition should be incurable and accompanied by severe, unrelenting, intolerable suffering. This particular criterion will be taken up a little later. Two other conditions are the existence of a meaningful doctor-patient relation and consultation. We have already discussed the difference between Hendin and Quill as to what would constitute a "meaningful" doctor-patient relation in circumstances like those of Diane. Hendin would make some efforts that Quill did not. Hendin is not presuming the rationality of suicide. Instead, he is bent on treating patients with suicidal ideation so as to prevent suicide. Let us examine this difference between Quill and Hendin from a clinical perspective to begin with.

Peter Sainsbury is a physician in England doing research in clinical psychiatry. After citing considerable research, Sainsbury makes these observations:

> It has therefore become our point of view that suicide falls squarely within the realm of community medicine and psychiatry; and prevention will depend on the capacity of the medical, psychiatric, and welfare personnel and on the willingness of the public health administrators to organize the social and psychiatric services in the light of the facts now available. The view that healthy people kill themselves, and justifiably so, if circumstances are sufficiently adverse, or that the individual should be "free" to decide his own fate is not tenable to us; the protection of the suicidal is as much a medical and community responsibility as any other cause of death against which prophylactic and therapeutic measures are available.[18]

Sainsbury urges that physicians be made aware of suicide as a preventable cause of death early on in their careers. He suggests further that psychiatrists educate general practitioners to accept suicide prevention "as a medical responsibility" and "to collaborate with the psychiatric services in dealing with the problem."[19] And, whereas Quill refers Diane to the Hemlock Society, Sainsbury would have physicians use the Samaritans to help in preventing suicide.

Quill mentions consultation as one of the criteria that should be met in

18. Peter Sainsbury, "Community Psychiatry," in S. Perlin, *A Handbook for the Study of Suicide* (New York: Oxford University Press, 1975), p. 173.
19. Sainsbury, "Community Psychiatry," p. 177.

decisions about aiding a patient to commit suicide. However, from Sainsbury's clinical perspective Quill has not properly met this criterion in the case of Diane. Once Diane expresses the wish to take her own life and have him assist her, a psychiatric consultation should have been sought.

But does Sainsbury's dictum really hold for dying patients in all circumstances? A recent psychiatric study notes the growth of movements such as the Voluntary Euthanasia Society in the United Kingdom and the Hemlock Society in the United States. Furthermore, the study points to the belief of these organizations that those who have painful, disfiguring, or disabling terminal illnesses should be encouraged to view suicide as a rational solution. The authors of this study cite research indicating that the numbers of suicides increase as a result of publicity, and further research indicating that suicides are almost always associated with mental disorders. The authors doubt that suicides stimulated by publicity are rational. What is more, they are convinced that depression is underdiagnosed and inadequately treated. With all of this in mind, they undertook a study of terminally ill patients who were competent and willing to give consent, and who experienced pain, severe disfigurement, and/or severe disability. They summarize their findings as follows:

> Among 44 terminally ill patients, the majority (N=34) had never wished death to come early. Of the remainder, three were or had been suicidal and seven more had desired early death. All the patients who had desired death were found to be suffering from clinical depressive illness.[20]

For obvious reasons, this study did not use "suicidal thinking" as a criterion for diagnosing depression. Although this is a small sample, this research, coupled with all the previous research, raises serious questions for the presumption that suicide is rational or ever can be.

But the belief of some philosophers and physicians that suicide can be rational does not tend to be swayed in the least by such research. Why is that?

Among philosophers, Richard B. Brandt gives one of the clearest accounts of why he thinks suicide should sometimes be regarded as rational. Normally, he regards it as reasonable that someone who takes a dim view of life on a given day considers that life may be better in days to come, even if that day is grim enough to make an individual despair of life. Brandt does believe, however, that when there are circumstances in which it is clear beyond any reasonable doubt that death has become preferable to life and will be un-

---

20. J. H. Brown et al., "Is It Normal for Terminally Ill Patients to Desire Death?" *American Journal of Psychiatry* 143, no. 2 (February 1986): 208.

til the end, "the rational thing is to act promptly."[21] "Let us not," he goes on to say, "pursue the question of whether it is rational for a person with a painful terminal illness to commit suicide; it is."[22] Brandt recognizes that individuals may harm others by taking their own lives and they should take this into account. He recognizes also that a state of depression clouds one's abilities to think straight, and therefore, if a decision to commit suicide is to be rational, it is best not to make it during a time of despair. However, if a decision has to be made, Brandt counsels someone contemplating suicide to "recall past reactions, in a normal frame of mind, to outcomes like those under assessment."[23] What makes a decision to commit suicide rational is that the circumstances warrant it. Death sometimes is a better prospect than continuing to live. That is exactly the stance taken by Quill and most recently by six prominent philosophers in a brief to the United States Supreme Court, arguing for declaring PAS to be a constitutional right.[24]

Hendin, the psychiatrist cited earlier, notes that what is currently called "rational suicide" by its proponents, draws on a concept of "balanced suicide," crafted by German philosophers early in this century. A "balanced suicide," Hendin tells us, was one in which

> Individuals assumed to be mentally unimpaired dispassionately took stock of their life situation and, having found it unacceptable or untenable and foreseeing no significant change for the better, decided to end their lives. Contemporary advocates see a close analogy between a rational decision for suicide and the decision of the directors of a firm to declare bankruptcy and get out of business.[25]

Hendin observes that the very idea that life can be assessed on a balance scale is a characteristic of suicidal people. Some of the most depressed patients spend years listing reasons why they should live to stack up against the many reasons they have for ending their lives. They have a tendency to state conditions that would make continuation of their lives intolerable, including the desire to exit if they cannot be in control. He concludes these observations

21. Richard B. Brandt, "The Morality and Rationality of Suicide," in S. Perlin, *A Handbook for the Study of Suicide,* p. 70.

22. Brandt, "The Morality and Rationality of Suicide," p. 70

23. Brandt, "The Morality and Rationality of Suicide," p. 72.

24. "Brief of Ronald Dworkin, Thomas Nagel, Robert Nozick, John Rawls, Thomas Scanlon, and Judith Jarvis Thomson as Amicus Curiae, in Support of Respondents," *Issues in Law and Medicine* 15, no. 2 (Fall 1999).

25. Hendin, "Seduced by Death," p. 134. See Hendin's footnote 43 for references to German philosophers and footnote 44 for references to contemporary advocates.

with what should give physicians like Quill some pause: "When a patient finds a doctor who shares the view that life is only worth living if certain conditions are met, the patient's rigidity is reinforced."[26]

But it is obvious that Quill, Brandt, and other physicians and philosophers favoring PAS are not convinced by Hendin's clinical observations. They do not link the idea that the worth of life can be calculated with being suicidal; it is a rational way of thinking. They regard it as primarily a mode of moral reasoning. Furthermore, they view making such assessments and acting on them as a basic human right that encompasses a "right to die."

It is instructive to examine the work of Alan Gewirth, one of the most persuasive defenders of human rights among contemporary philosophers. Gewirth contends that every human being has a right to life. Although the right to life is not absolute, in that self-defense and violence against oppression can be justified, "all innocent persons have an absolute right not to be the intended victims of a homicidal project."[27] Yet, at the same time, Gewirth argues for a right to commit suicide, that is, a right to make oneself the intended "victim of a homicidal project." However, he would not consider the one who rationally and freely commits suicide a "victim" but rather as one who is claiming and acting upon the basic right to freedom enjoyed by all human beings. How does Gewirth seek to make his case? To begin with,

> human rights . . . are rights of every human being to the necessary conditions of human action, i.e., those conditions that must be fulfilled if human action is to be possible either at all or with general chances of success in achieving the purposes for which humans act.[28]

He identifies freedom and well-being, including life, as "the procedural and substantive necessary conditions of acting for any purposes either at all or with any chances of success."[29] These are the "objects" of our rights, what we have a right to, namely freedom and well-being. It would be a logical contradiction to deny the necessity of freedom and well-being for action. Having argued that the "objects" of human rights are the necessary conditions of human action, Gewirth believes he has proof that it is freedom and well-being that are claimed as human rights.

26. Hendin, "Seduced by Death," p. 134.

27. Alan Gewirth, *Human Rights: Essays on Justification and Applications* (Chicago: University of Chicago Press, 1982), p. 233. By describing a right as "absolute," Gewirth means that it cannot be overridden in any circumstances, and so can never be justifiably "infringed," and must be "fulfilled" without any exceptions (p. 219).

28. Gewirth, *Human Rights*, p. 3.

29. Gewirth, *Human Rights*, p. 4.

In elaborating some further reasons why human rights should be based on the necessary conditions of human action, he claims that

> all the human rights, those of well-being as well as of freedom, have as their aim that each person have rational autonomy in the sense of being a self-controlling, self-developing agent who can relate to other persons on a basis of mutual respect and cooperation, in contrast to being a dependent passive recipient of the actions of others.[30]

Gewirth is aware that actualizing rights sometimes requires assistance from others. But such aid should not be for the purpose of reinforcing or increasing dependence, but rather for supporting persons in the "control of their own lives" and in the pursuit of their own purposes without being dominated or harmed by others. "In this way," Gewirth asserts, "agency is the metaphysical and moral basis of human dignity."[31] It should be noted that, on this view, the loss of one's abilities to act and a state of increased dependence entail a loss of dignity. Being in control is, as in Quill, an expression of dignity, and being in control of the time and manner of one's dying is a way to achieve death with dignity, devoid of a state of dependence and of greatly diminished powers to act.

But how can suicide be considered a right, when the freedom to undertake it puts an end to all possibilities to act, to freedom and life, and hence is an act that abolishes these basic rights? Why not conclude that abolishing these rights is a violation of them? The first clue lies in Gewirth's understanding of the right to freedom. It is, for a recipient of action, first of all, "a right to be let alone by others until and unless he unforcedly consents to undergo their action."[32] This means that people have "a sphere of personal autonomy and privacy."[33] Coercion or harm may be necessary to protect agents from the harm others might inflict or from violating the freedom of others. The freedom of individuals may also be restricted in order to prevent agents from seriously harming themselves or to prevent them from giving up their own dispositional freedom; but coercion or interference for these reasons should be temporary.[34] We now have all of the ingredients of Gewirth's justification for suicide. Committing suicide, which harms only the one committing it, is

---

30. Gewirth, *Human Rights*, p. 5.

31. Gewirth, *Human Rights*, p. 5.

32. Alan Gewirth, *Reason and Morality* (Chicago: University of Chicago Press, 1978), p. 256.

33. Gewirth, *Reason and Morality*, p. 256.

34. Gewirth, *Reason and Morality*, p. 271.

in the sphere of private, autonomous action. Efforts to prevent a suicide should be temporary lest that agent's right to freedom be violated by refusing to respect the right to exercise one's right to autonomy and privacy. Even though suicide ends one's life and freedom, the act itself is an expression of freedom as an act that is free of the interference of others.

Although Gewirth posits a moral responsibility to save and protect human lives, including a "duty to rescue," he does not posit a moral responsibility to protect one's own life, provided that no one is harmed by taking one's own life. In all of this, Gewirth is making some implicit assumptions about human nature, about what kind of selves we are and what kinds of relationships naturally obtain among human beings and their communities. For Gewirth, when we act freely, without interference, we seek goods for ourselves. Well-being and life are necessary for this quest but whether we regard life as a good is a matter of choice and a choice we ought to be free to make for ourselves. To be prevented from choosing whether to be or not to be is to have our dignity as human beings violated. The freedom not to be interfered with is the moral right that no person should give up and no person presumably would want to give up; the right to live, however, persons may reasonably give up. Gewirth has made life a sub-category of well-being and absolutized the right to non-interference in acts regarded as private. This is a move made in American law. I refer to the dictum that "the right to life has come to mean the right to enjoy life, — the right to be let alone."[35] It was this right also that was cited by the Ninth Circuit Court of Appeals in its decision in 1996 to declare a constitutional right to PAS, a decision, however, that was reversed by the U.S. Supreme Court in 1997.[36]

Gewirth has adopted Mills's egoistic hedonism that has human beings seeking their own happiness or well-being. He has dropped the Hobbesian and Lockean view of our natural inclinations as human beings, a view also found in American law. Hobbes and Locke regarded every human being as naturally inclined toward self-preservation, and that meant the preservation of one's own life. For them, it was irrational to destroy one's own life; it was rational to give up freedom to preserve it. That willingness to surrender some of one's freedom in order to gain the power of a sovereign to defend one's life, was at the core of the social contract and its legitimation of sovereignty. The right to life was not to be and could not be surrendered for it was a natural,

---

35. See Mary Ann Glendon, *Rights Talk: The Impoverishment of Political Discourse* (New York: Free Press, 1991), pp. 47-75.

36. *Compassion in Dying v. State of Washington*, 79 F. 3rd 790 (9th Cir. 1996) overturned by *Washington v. Glucksberg*, 117 S.Ct. 2258 (1997).

inalienable human possession. Gewirth does not tie rationality, dignity, and self-control to retaining one's right to life, but to being an agent, free to control one's own life, without being subjected to interference in one's quest for happiness, and without being subjected to harm from others.

The philosopher Immanuel Kant rejects this sort of thinking on suicide, and one of his major arguments hinges on an understanding of human nature at odds with that of Gewirth. As Kant says, "We shrink in horror from suicide because all nature seeks its own preservation."[37] Preserving one's life is an expression of one's humanity. Humanity in one's own person is inviolable; it is never, for Kant, permissible to commit suicide. An act of suicide makes a thing of oneself and in setting out to act in this way, one ceases to be human: "The role of morality does not admit of it under any conditions because it degrades human nature below the level of animal nature and so destroys it."[38]

Whereas Gewirth proclaims a moral right to commit suicide and sees human dignity attained by not letting anyone rob an agent of the freedom to exercise this right freely claimed, Kant sees suicide under all circumstances as a paradigm case of completely losing one's dignity as a human being. With different conceptions of what constitutes our humanity and of what qualities humans naturally possess, we make different choices with regard to what is moral and what is rational. And so what is rational and dignified for Gewirth is both irrational and undignified for Hobbes and Kant when it comes to suicide. What divides Quill's clinical perspectives from that of Hendin and Sainsbury are their assumptions about what to expect from human nature. In Quill's case, wishing for suicide can be rational. For Hendin and Sainsbury, wishing for suicide means that individuals need to be treated for whatever is distorting their ability to think rationally. Empirical findings are generated and interpreted through these different lenses. Unless these underlying premises are addressed, the participants in the debate over the rationality of suicide will not be impressed with one another's arguments or data. Indeed, that is the present reality.

But Gewirth's conception of selfhood not only affects what he regards as human rights but also what he regards as the substance and structure of moral life and of the human relations comprising that structure. Gewirth depicts the self in a way that supposes that each of us as human agents can logically and experientially choose whether and to what degree we are connected to others. But no one came to be and to be sustained without parental nurture and com-

---

37. Immanuel Kant, *Lectures on Ethics* (New York: Harper & Row, 1983), p. 150.
38. Kant, *Lectures on Ethics*, p. 152.

munal protection. There is a whole network of moral responsibilities in the form of human relations that make life possible at all. Gewirth supposes that individuals can achieve a form of isolation or disconnectedness such that harms we do to ourselves, including self-destruction, are not harmful to others, or at least should not be viewed as such. He does not even address the kind of harm that occurs when others and whole communities are encouraged to decrease their inhibitions against killing, and their proclivity to nurture and protect lives, their own and others. The English poet John Donne differs sharply from Gewirth in how he views our relations to one another as human beings. In his work *Devotions,* he maintains that no one is an island and every person's death diminishes him. So close is this tie to another person's death that Donne concludes his portrayal of it with these much quoted lines: "And therefore never send to know for whom the bell tolls. It tolls for thee." Donne is reflecting what is characteristic of the view of human nature found in the Jewish and Christian traditions: We are naturally social and we have the natural ability and proclivity to be morally responsible for our relations to one another, indeed to love one another, even when strangers. And, love of neighbor is a summary of the moral law that includes the prohibition against killing.

The debate, then, over whether suicide is rational and socially justifiable is carried on, at least currently, without attention to the theories of human nature and human relatedness that actually divide the disputants, and that incline them to be utterly unpersuaded by one another's arguments and empirical observations. In Chapter Three, I will argue that there is a way beyond these particular disputes by attention to the moral requisites of agential and communal life.

Going Beyond the Alleviation of Suffering by Eliminating or Avoiding It Altogether

As we have already indicated in this chapter, hospice care began, and continues presently, to meet the needs that some think can only be met through ending one's life with a physician's assistance, by providing excellent relief of pain and other symptoms. In his arguments against the resort to PAS, the noted physician Edmund Pellegrino recognizes that pain and suffering, and the fear of lack of control, should be addressed, especially now when medical technology has the power to prolong life:

> There is nothing in the Christian tradition that binds patients or physicians to pursue futile and excessively burdensome treatment, i.e., treatments

whose benefits are disproportionate to the burdens it imposes — physical, emotional, or fiscal. Patients may reach a point, therefore, in the natural history of their illnesses at which further treatment serves no beneficial purpose. . . . Refusal or discontinuance of treatment with little or no effectiveness or benefit . . . does not mean abandonment. On the contrary, it enjoins and entails an obligation for more efforts at palliative care, hospice, or home support.[39]

Quill probably is aware that hospice, and palliative care generally, are highly effective in providing relief for pain and suffering, as noted in the literature cited at footnote 39. But to him, hospice and palliative care, however exquisite, are not sufficient for some patients. Some patients, however small the percentage, will be forced to choose between pain, so that they may be conscious and interact with others, and sedation, without these possibilities. Quill describes a woman, Mrs. B, who lived for ten days sedated before dying. Her friends and family "found the experience deeply disturbing," and, to Quill, forcing Mrs. B "into a medically induced twilight zone so she could then die of natural causes seemed macabre." And, Quill adds, doing so is "cruel and absurd."[40] The compassionate response, and therefore ethical response, to Mrs. B's pain and suffering would have been PAS.[41]

In the case of Mrs. B and the case of Diane, Quill advocates to go beyond the *relief* of pain and suffering. Indeed, he went beyond putting an end to suffering. In the case of Diane, the resort to PAS was a response to the *possibility* that Diane's suffering *could* result in requiring her to choose between pain and sedation. Her fear that comfort care could reach such a point, and her aversions to being "out of control," "bed-bound," "totally dependent," or confused, "waiting for death" could only be satisfactorily addressed by helping her to end her life even before she suffered.[42] In short, Quill is engaging in PAS *not just to eliminate suffering but to avoid it.* Why go through some of the inevitable suffering of the dying process, at the very least the deterioration of

39. Edmund D. Pellegrino, "Euthanasia and Assisted Suicide," in John F. Kilner et al., eds., *Dignity and Dying,* p. 114. Palliative care can be highly effective though it should be used more than it is. For example, see the New York State Task Force on Life and the Law, *When Death Is Sought: Assisted Suicide and Euthanasia in the Medical Context,* May 1994; Kathleen M. Foley, "Doctoring the Doctor," *Hastings Center Report* 24, no. 3 (May-June, 1994): 45-46; and Shannon Brownlee and Joanne M. Schrof, "Effective Pain Treatments Already Exist. Why Aren't Doctors Using Them?" *U.S. News and World Report,* March 17, 1997, pp. 54-67.

40. Quill, *Death and Dignity,* pp. 111-12.

41. Quill, *Death and Dignity,* p. 140.

42. Quill, *Death and Dignity,* p. 105.

one's physical and mental powers, if one can avoid it? As Quill says, prolongation of the dying process might have a purpose for some; for others "it is meaningless and even cruel."[43] What should be prevented is a "continued meaningless existence with no escape."[44] Indeed, Quill considers it among the objectives of medicine to prolong a "*meaningful* life" and to *humanize* the "process of dying."[45] To meet this latter objective, PAS is necessary in some instances.

Pellegrino is among those who argue that PAS is not necessary, and just as pain should be treated, so should suffering. Pain and suffering are not the same.[46] Suffering, when it is a response to a physically noxious stimulus that causes pain, is subjective. There are reasons other than pain for suffering, such as

> feelings of guilt at being a burden to others, mental depression, alienation from the world of the healthy, fear of the process of dying, spiritual confusion, the dissolution of life plans, as well as the attitudes of care-givers, friends or family whose fear and distaste for the sight of suffering will be perceived by the suffering person . . . [and] add to the desire to be rid even of life, to escape.[47]

All of these modes of suffering can and should be addressed without resort to PAS. In fact, the kind of negative reaction Quill exhibits to individuals who are suffering in certain ways, helpless and dependent, is one reason to bar physicians from favoring PAS, for such negative reactions to the dying process add to, or stimulate, suffering it may be possible to alleviate or even eliminate.

But Quill is not moved by such entreaties to abandon PAS as an additional method of preventing and eliminating suffering. He, and those who share his views, also will not be persuaded by data that support the effectiveness of treating pain and suffering. There are two major reasons for this.

First, when Quill describes PAS as *humanizing* the dying process, as noted above, we once more encounter the assumption that "being in control," avoiding unhappiness and ending life in order to accomplish these purposes, are at the heart of living in accord with one's humanity. Quill shares the view of human nature espoused by Gewirth, discussed earlier. Like Gewirth, he

43. Quill, *Death and Dignity*, p. 106.
44. Quill, *Death and Dignity*, p. 25.
45. Quill, *Death and Dignity*, p. 25.
46. See, for example, Eric Cassell, *The Nature of Suffering* (New York: Oxford University Press, 1991).
47. Pellegrino, "Euthanasia and Assisted Suicide," p. 114.

does not posit any natural continuous inclination to preserve one's life. In-deed, also like Gewirth, he regards taking one's own life as something individ-uals are free to do when there are circumstances such that choosing to do so can be considered to be rational. Arguments for an alternative view of human nature and suicide will be presented in Chapters Three and Four.

There is, however, another reason that Quill is not persuaded that PAS should not be one of the medical responses to suffering. For Pellegrino and like-minded individuals, PAS is unethical regardless of whether one is moved by compassion to offer it. Yet, Pellegrino and many others, also moved by compassion, advocate that "there should be no hesitance to use analgesics and other agents optimally and in sufficient dose even if the non-intended side effect is to accelerate dying."[48] But Quill's retort is to claim that there is no significant moral difference between hastening death through comfort care and doing so by means of PAS. If one is willing to give ethical approval to hastening death through pain relief and through the refusal of life-sustaining technology, such as respiration, then there is no justifiable reason to disap-prove hastening death through the use of PAS. If comfort care can be rational, so can PAS. Furthermore, that the wishes of patients are subject to being in-fluenced or even coerced by others, and subject to change for a variety of rea-sons, is as true of the wishes for comfort care as it is of wishes for PAS. In both instances, abuse is possible, and when death is hastened, abuse can be equally fatal. It is necessary, therefore, to take on the very critical question as to whether there are morally significant differences between PAS and palliative care. That is the task of the chapter that now follows.

---

48. Pellegrino, "Euthanasia and Assisted Suicide," p. 114.

CHAPTER TWO

Physician-Assisted Suicide versus Comfort-Only Care: Do They Differ Morally in Significant Ways?

There is no doubt about the importance of addressing the question as to whether PAS and comfort-only care differ morally in significant ways. The argument that they do not determined the decision of the Second Circuit Court of Appeals to declare PAS, in certain circumstances, to be a constitutional right.[1] Indeed, in this decision, *Quill v. Vacco*, Dr. Quill, whose views we examined extensively in Chapter One, is quoted approvingly on this very matter:

> The removal of a life support system that directly results in the patient's death requires the direct involvement by the doctor as well as other medical personnel. When such patients are mentally competent they are consciously choosing death as preferable to life under the circumstances that they are forced to live. Their doctors do a careful clinical assessment, including a full exploration of the patient's prognosis, mental competence to make such decisions, and the treatment alternatives to stopping treatment. It is legally and ethically permitted for physicians to actively assist patients to die who are dependent on life-sustaining treatment. . . . Unfortunately, some dying patients who are in agony that can no longer be relieved, yet are not dependent on life-sustaining treatment, have no such options under current legal restrictions. It seems unfair, discriminatory, and inhumane to deprive some dying patients of such vital choices because of arbitrary elements of their condition, which determine whether they are on life-sustaining treatment that can be stopped.[2]

1. *Quill v. Vacco*, 80 F3rd. 716 (2nd Cir., 1996).
2. *Quill v. Vacco*, 721.

That the Second Court of Appeals accepts Quill's argument as cited above is obvious in the following passage:

> ... the writing of a prescription to hasten death, after consultation with a patient, involves a far less active role for the physician than is required in bringing about death through asphyxiation, starvation and/or dehydration. Withdrawal of life support requires physicians or those acting at their discretion physically to remove equipment and often to administer palliative drugs which may themselves contribute to death. The ending of life by these means is nothing more or less than assisted suicide. It simply cannot be said that those mentally competent, terminally ill persons who seek to hasten death but whose treatment does not include life support are treated equally.[3]

This alleged inequality occurs in law and, therefore, the prohibition violates the Equal Protection Clause of the Fourteenth Amendment, requiring that the law equally protect individuals who are similar to one another in relevant ways.

In reversing the decision of the Second Circuit Court of Appeals, the U.S. Supreme Court directly disputed the Court's assertion as quoted immediately above:

> On their faces, neither the assisted-suicide ban nor the law permitting patients to refuse medical treatment treats anyone differently from anyone else or draws any distinctions between persons. *Everyone,* regardless of physical condition, is entitled, if competent, to refuse unwanted lifesaving medical treatment; *no one* is permitted to assist a suicide. Generally laws that apply evenhandedly to all unquestionably comply with equal protection. . . . This Court disagrees with the Second Circuit's submission that ending or refusing lifesaving medical treatment "is nothing more or less than assisted suicide." The distinction between letting a patient die and making that patient die is important, logical, rational, and well established. It comports with fundamental legal principles of causation . . . and intent . . . and has been widely recognized and endorsed in the medical profession, the state courts, and the overwhelming majority of state legislatures, which, like New York's, have permitted the former while prohibiting the latter. . . . Logic and contemporary practice support New York's judgment that the two acts are different, and New York may therefore, consistent with the Constitution, treat them differently.[4]

3. *Quill v. Vacco*, 729.
4. *Vacco v. Quill*, 117 S.Ct. 2293 (1997), 2295.

For the present, then, the distinction between PAS and modes of comfort care that may shorten life is enshrined in American constitutional law and state legislatures, with the exception of Oregon.[5] However, given the denial of this distinction in the Second Circuit, and by eight of eleven judges on the Ninth Circuit Court of Appeals,[6] the future course of American constitutional law cannot with certainty be predicted. Likewise, given Oregon's move toward PAS, future legislation cannot with certainty be predicted. Furthermore, what happens to this distinction both reflects and shapes the moral outlook and behavior of individuals and communities. For all these reasons, I turn to consider the merit of arguments for and against maintaining the current, legally recognized differences between PAS and comfort-only care that may have the effect of hastening death. For such an analysis, I will examine sources that provide nuanced philosophical arguments beyond those found in the courts. But first the terminology that I use needs to be clarified.

Some Critical Conceptual Issues

I have been using the expression "comfort-only care" and distinguishing it from PAS. By comfort-only care, I mean that the care being given a patient is aimed at the relief of pain and suffering, and all other possible interventions are evaluated from the perspective of what they contribute to the relief of pain and suffering. The resort to comfort-only care occurs when curative efforts are no longer regarded as efficacious. Whether all other life-sustaining interventions are to be refused, whether withheld or withdrawn, becomes a matter of evaluating how burdensome they are, relative to what benefits they may have. These decisions with respect to life-sustaining treatment not only have comfort in view, they may also seek to prolong life even while dying of a terminal disease, in order to accomplish certain purposes, such as taking leave of loved ones or finishing some project, given, of course, that a patient's condition allows for whatever energy and communicative abilities are necessary for such purposes. But pain relief can hasten death, and the refusal of life-sustaining modalities, such as a respirator, can quickly end life. Such examples raise the question as to whether decisions of comfort-only care that clearly hasten death are in any way significantly different from decisions to

---

5. "The Oregon Death with Dignity Act" is reprinted in Margaret P. Battin, Rosamond Rhodes, and Anita Silvers, eds., *Physician-Assisted Suicide: Expanding the Debate* (New York: Routledge, 1998), Appendix D.

6. *Compassion in Dying v. State of Washington,* 79 F. 3rd 790 (9th Cir. 1996).

request PAS, or even euthanasia, when curative efforts have been justifiably abandoned and the focus is on ending pain and suffering.

Suicide is the voluntary and intentional killing of oneself.[7] The term "voluntary" is essential to attributing the act that ends life to the agent whose life it is. The term "intentional" is used to contrast suicide as an act from an act that would be properly deemed to be accidental, as in the case of a gun assumed to be unloaded that discharges and kills the one who pressed the trigger. This terminology does not exclude the possibility that some or all acts of ending one's life may be done in a psychological state of depression such that, from a psychological point of view, the act is not rationally or totally "voluntary" in every sense of the word, and not rationally or totally "intentional" in every sense of that word. *Physician-assisted suicide* (PAS) occurs when a physician, knowing that the patient's intention is to commit suicide, provides the means used to carry it out, means such as information, prescriptions, or a "suicide machine."

Euthanasia, in its original meaning, referred to a "good" death. It has come to mean "mercy killing." A mercy killing takes place when someone motivated by compassion intentionally and actively kills someone to end that individual's suffering. *Voluntary euthanasia* is carried out at the request of the individual whose life is ended; *involuntary euthanasia* is carried out without the request or consent of the competent individual whose life is ended; *nonvoluntary euthanasia* is carried out on incompetent individuals.

Discussions of PAS and euthanasia usually take up the distinction between *active* and *passive* euthanasia. The term "active euthanasia" is actually just another way to describe what has been defined as "euthanasia" in the paragraph immediately above. I will use the term "euthanasia" to refer only to "active euthanasia." "Passive euthanasia" is used to describe situations in which life-sustaining treatments are withheld or withdrawn from a terminally ill patient, allowing the individual to die naturally.[8] The expressions "letting die" and "allowing to die" have also been applied to these same circumstances. I prefer employing "comfort-only care" to refer to these kinds of situations. Since "euthanasia" has come to be associated with "mercy killing,"

---

7. See Robert D. Orr, "The Physician-Assisted Suicide: Is It Ever Justified?" in T. J. Demy and G. P. Stewart, eds., *Suicide: A Christian Response* (Grand Rapids: Kregel, 1998), ch. 4.

8. Dying naturally may be a somewhat ambiguous term in this context. It is intended to refer to the fact that the individuals who die do so as a result of their conditions and not as a result of some act intended to end their life. If the withholding or withdrawing of treatment is done expressly for the purpose of ending a patient's life, it is morally akin to active euthanasia.

it can be confusing as a description of situations that include, for example, refusing an experimental treatment that promises to prolong life but which could very likely also cause the death of a patient. What is being refused is high-risk intervention with its burdensome side effects in order to pursue other activities free of such risks and burdens. Comfort-only care appropriately depicts such situations. The terms "passive," "letting," and "allowing" are also less than satisfactory ways to describe how a physician is expected to relate to a patient who is dying. Patients who are dying need care, or assistance for obtaining care, such as nursing care at home, from the physician(s) who have judged that they are indeed beyond a cure. Comfort-only care is a clearer way to refer to these practices in medicine, since relief of pain and suffering is regarded as an obligation of physicians irrespective of what other medical interventions may or may not be involved when such an obligation exists toward a given patient.

Allowing to die or *letting die* are often considered to be morally different from killing. But correctly labeling an act as "allowing to die" does not tell us whether the act is morally justified. If, for example, an individual whose life could have been saved in an emergency room is knowingly and deliberately allowed to die, such inaction would be morally akin to an unjustified killing, given the moral and legal obligations to treat in such circumstances. (In this instance I am assuming that the time, resources, and medical personnel are all sufficient to save that individual's life.) At the same time, killing in defense of a life is generally accepted as morally and legally justified. A physician who had to use such force to defend herself against a patient turned violent that the patient died from the struggle may be said to have killed that patient, but justifiably, albeit tragically, under those circumstances. Resorting to comfort-only care also may sometimes be morally akin to killing if, for example, it is knowingly done for a patient who is judged to be curable by conventionally accepted medical means, who is not properly informed of that fact, or for whom no efforts to seek consent for treatment have been made.

Therefore, the question to which we now attend, the question as to whether there is a moral difference between comfort-only care and PAS, is more precisely a question as to whether comfort-only care can sometimes be morally justified whereas PAS never can be. As we will see, that discussion will require attention to euthanasia as well as PAS.

Arguments That Equate Some Instances of PAS and Euthanasia with Morally Justifiable Comfort-Only Care: An Analysis

In the fourth edition of their text in bioethics, Tom Beauchamp and James Childress have argued in favor of PAS as a public policy, and argued as well on behalf of the moral acceptability of PAS and euthanasia under exceptional and highly circumscribed circumstances.[9] A critical element in drawing these conclusions is to argue that

> If competent patients have a legal and moral right to refuse treatment that involves health professionals in implementing their decision and bringing about their deaths, we have a reason to suppose they have a similar right to request the assistance of willing physicians to help them control the conditions under which they die. Assuming that omission of treatment is justified by the principles of respect for autonomy and nonmaleficence, cannot the same form of justification be extended to physicians prescribing barbiturates needed by seriously ill patients, and possibly to physician-administered lethal injections?[10]

Beauchamp and Childress note that this argument points to an apparent inconsistency: Patients have a right based on their autonomy, in grim circumstances, to refuse treatment so as to bring about their deaths, but they are denied such a right, in equally grim circumstances, to arrange for their death by mutual agreement between themselves and their physicians. The authors believe that the need to exercise the right to have one's life ended with the help of a physician involves only a small percentage of patients because of the great strides in pain management, improved environments for patients, and the existence of hospice to care for the dying. But this does not, in this view, suffice for all conditions in which patients find themselves. And Beauchamp and Childress add,

> in any event there are significant questions about autonomy rights for patients. If a right exists to stop a machine that sustains life, through an arrangement involving mutual agreement with a physician, why is there not the same right to stop the machine that *is* one's life by an arrangement with a physician?[11]

9. Tom L. Beauchamp and James F. Childress, *Principles of Biomedical Ethics,* 4th ed. (New York: Oxford University Press, 1994). As indicated on p. 7, n. 15, the 5th edition came out too late to be included in this book. However, the authors have not changed their position on PAS and euthanasia or the arguments put forth, though they are stated more concisely.

10. Beauchamp and Childress, *Principles of Biomedical Ethics,* p. 226.

11. Beauchamp and Childress, *Principles of Biomedical Ethics,* p. 226.

It is important to note that Beauchamp and Childress are not simply equating every act of refusing treatment with acts that are intended to end life. A patient may choose to discontinue a treatment that is futile to prevent death. In an example they provide, Beauchamp and Childress describe a situation in which an individual will live for one month more with or without continuing dialysis. When the patient in this case elects to stop dialysis treatments in order to be at home with loved ones, free of the machine and the hospital, there is no suicidal intent as some have argued.[12] Suicide is the wrong category to apply and so then is PAS because death will result, with or without treatment, from untreatable conditions that are not arranged by the patient for the purpose of ending life: "This is what we might call a 'pure' refusal case that lacks all suicidal intent."[13] But refusals of treatment "are instances of suicide whenever the agent specifically arranges the conditions to bring about death."[14] Since, in the view of Beauchamp and Childress, these refusals are generally morally and legally accepted under certain "grim" circumstances, there is no justifiable reason to ban PAS and even voluntary euthanasia under similarly "grim" circumstances. The autonomy of patients should be honored in both ways of choosing to die.

There is a long-accepted argument, the rule of double effect (RDE), that refusals of treatment that are, or should be, morally accepted and legally recognized are never instances of suicide or anything morally equivalent. Refusals of treatment that knowingly result in death are not viewed as acts of suicide. For example, in cases in which patients are terminally ill, a physician's providing of pain relief that has a substantial probability of shortening life is not considered PAS, and unlike PAS is morally justifiable. In these same circumstances, providing a lethal injection (euthanasia) to end pain is regarded as wrongfully killing the patient, and the patient is wrongfully requesting such actions. What is morally justifiable is the provision of medication with the intention of relieving pain, without in any way intending to hasten death. If no intention of ending life with a known lethal effect exists in such a case, this act is morally justified because it does not directly and intentionally harm (kill) an innocent individual.

Beauchamp and Childress find fault with a key element in the RDE. "Adherents of the RDE need an account of intentional actions and intended effects of action (intentionally causing or allowing) that properly distin-

---

12. Beauchamp and Childress, *Principles of Biomedical Ethics*, p. 224. See especially the quotation of and reference to the philosopher Dan Brock.
13. Beauchamp and Childress, *Principles of Biomedical Ethics*, p. 224.
14. Beauchamp and Childress, *Principles of Biomedical Ethics*, p. 224.

guishes them from nonintentional actions and unintended effects (foresee-ably causing or allowing)."[15] This the RDE cannot provide. Beauchamp and Childress begin their reasons for this claim by calling attention to a view that is widely shared in an otherwise controversial literature on intention: Inten-tional actions are characterized by an agent's plan, one that contains some representation of the means and ends being proposed. For an action to be deemed intentional, it has to be in accord with the agent's conception of how it was planned to be performed. Using "a model of intentionality based on what is *willed* rather than what is *wanted*," Beauchamp and Childress assert that "intentional actions and intentional effects include any action and any effect willed in accordance with a plan, including tolerated as well as wanted effects."[16] Given this conception of intention, there is no viable distinction between what is intended and what is only foreseeable:

> Thus a person who knowingly and voluntarily acts to bring about an effect brings about that effect intentionally. The effect is intended, although the person did not desire it, did not will it for its own sake, or did not intend it as the goal of the action.[17]

This way of understanding intentional actions means that physicians who have pain relief as their goal, and whose interventions for that purpose also hasten death, have, at the same time, intentionally served as a causal agent in the deaths of such patients. If killing someone is described as causing someone's death, then one can view these deaths as examples of physicians killing patients. Legally they are not described in this way, nor do Beauchamp and Childress advocate that they be described in this way. Rather, what they advocate is that hastening death by means of pain relief, or refusal of life-sustaining treatment in the circumstances now generally sanctioned morally and legally, should be recognized as no different morally from hastening death by PAS or euthanasia: all of these actions are morally the same — they cause the death of patients in very dire circumstances and they arrange their deaths through mutually agreed upon procedures. It should be noted that Beauchamp and Childress advocate the legalization of PAS though they would not oppose legalizing euthanasia.

Beauchamp and Childress have not resorted to the simpler arguments

15. Beauchamp and Childress, *Principles of Biomedical Ethics*, p. 208.

16. Beauchamp and Childress, *Principles of Biomedical Ethics*, p. 209. See pages 206-11 for a full description and critique of the RDE. For significant elaborations and uses of the RDE see the references cited for footnote 41, at page 252.

17. Beauchamp and Childress, *Principles of Biomedical Ethics*, p. 209.

of some consequentialists — that the practices they equate are morally indistinguishable because they both have the same effect, namely that the patient's life is foreshortened. They have retained the very important concept of intention, a concept that courts use to judge, among other things, how culpable someone is for having killed another individual and for distinguishing intentional from accidentally caused deaths. In *Vacco v. Quill*, the U.S. Supreme Court cited some of the uses of intent in the law:

> The law has long used actors' intent or purpose to distinguish between two acts that may have the same result.... ("[T]he ... common law of homicide often distinguishes ... between a person who knows that another person will be killed as a result of his conduct and a person who acts with the specific purpose of taking another's life") ... (distinctions based on intent are "universal and persistent in mature systems of law"). [All references have been omitted.][18]

The Court concluded this paragraph with the language and reasoning of the RDE as embedded in law: "... the law distinguishes actions taken 'because of' a given end from actions taken 'in spite of' their unintended but foreseen consequences."[19] The Court finds that this same mode of reasoning, in law and by the medical profession, compels them to reject the claim of the Second Circuit Court of Appeals in *Quill v. Vacco* (1994) that ending or refusing life-sustaining treatment "is nothing more or less than assisted suicide."[20] Rehnquist, writing for a unanimous court, and arguing on the basis of legal decisions and medical sources, began by noting that "when a patient refuses life sustaining medical treatment, he dies from an under-lying fatal disease or pathology; but if a patient ingests lethal medication prescribed by a physician, he is killed by that medication."[21] Rehnquist cited legal decisions that include the removal of feeding tubes among the life-sustaining treatments that should not be equated with intending the death of the patient. Among other citations, Rehnquist quoted the American Medical Association on Ethical and Judicial Affairs: "When a life-sustaining treatment is declined, the patient dies primarily because of an underlying disease."[22]

Moving from considerations of causation to considerations of intent, Rehnquist observed that physicians who withdraw or honor a patient's re-

18. *Vacco v. Quill*, 2299.
19. *Vacco v. Quill*, 2299.
20. *Quill v. Vacco*, 729.
21. *Vacco v. Quill*, 2298.
22. *Vacco v. Quill*, 2298.

fusal to initiate life-sustaining medical interventions, purposefully intend, or may so intend, only to respect the patient's wishes and,

> to cease doing useless and futile or degrading things to the patient when [the patient] no longer stands to benefit from them. . . . The same is true when a doctor provides aggressive palliative care; in some cases, painkilling drugs may hasten a patient's death, but the physician's purpose and intent is, or may be only to ease his patient's pain. A doctor who assists a suicide, however, "must necessarily and indubitably intend primarily that the patient be made dead." . . . Similarly, a patient who commits suicide with a doctor's aid necessarily has the specific intent to end his or her own life, while a patient who refuses or discontinues treatment might not . . . [but] may instead "fervently wish to live, but to do so free of unwanted technology, surgery, or drugs."[23]

Clearly, jurists would not be persuaded by this whole line of reasoning found in law, and some are not, if they rejected the RDE for the reasons offered by Beauchamp and Childress. But have Beauchamp and Childress defined intent and described causation in such a way that Rehnquist's reasoning as quoted above has to be rejected? I think not.

Arguments That Specify How PAS and Euthanasia Differ Morally from Comfort-Only Care

To begin with, I find that Beauchamp and Childress have described intent and causation in a plausible but partially misleading way. They concluded that "intentional actions and intentional effects include any action and any effect willed in accordance with the plan, including tolerated as well as wanted effects."[24] This means that what Rehnquist, in accord with the RDE, calls "foreseen consequences" are to be viewed as intended. One certainly can use intention in that way. But it is misleading simply to describe physicians as causing death when, through increasing pain relief or withdrawing some type of life support, they foresee and tolerate the death of their patients. Physicians cannot, by willing it to be so, assure that a given disease will or will not be fatal. Patients properly diagnosed as terminal will die because of the effects of their disease upon their bodies, unless someone kills them outright by the use of means known to be lethal.

23. *Vacco v. Quill,* 2298-99.
24. Beauchamp and Childress, *Principles of Biomedical Ethics,* p. 209.

Beauchamp and Childress are not wrong to view physicians as causal agents when they create circumstances that will foreseeably affect the *timing* of a patient's death. But unless physicians use known lethal means to affect the timing of a death, it is not correct to describe them as causing the deaths of terminally ill patients. In such instances, fatal diseases are functioning to bring about deaths physicians are helpless to prevent.

The RDE, then, remains relevant with respect to detecting moral differences between intending comfort-only care and intending death. Indeed Beauchamp and Childress do not dismiss every aspect of the RDE. They employ one of its "rules" in deciding what actions are morally justifiable. I refer to the principle of "proportionality" that would justifiably allow a harmful effect "only if a proportionately weighty good will probably be brought about."[25] In other words, one weighs the relation between burdens and benefits to help determine whether an act is morally justified. I want to begin my argument on this very point but to describe this consideration in a somewhat different way.

The late eminent twentieth-century moral philosopher, W. D. Ross, observed that most actions are morally complex.[26] They are morally complex in the sense that they have more than one right- or wrong-making characteristic. One example would be an act that is done for the sake of saving an accident victim, which act is at the same time an act that breaks a promise to meet a friend for dinner at a particular time. Instead of analyzing this as a case in which to apply the RDE, which would be applicable, Ross speaks of saving a life as the most right act in the circumstances. The act in question is right insofar as it is an act of saving a life but wrong insofar as it is an act of breaking a promise. To claim that saving a life is the most right thing to do and, as Ross would also claim, one's actual duty in the circumstances, is to consider saving a life as having more moral weight than keeping the particular promise in question. If, however, breaking a promise would result in the death of the one to whom the promise was made, Ross would view keeping this promise and saving this life as the most right action relative to saving someone else's life for two reasons: (1) keeping the promise satisfies two right-making characteristics; (2) non-maleficence, refraining from harm, is generally more stringent (weighty) than beneficence, doing something good for another. For Ross, the rightness of acts depends upon what kinds of actions they are. Thus, refraining from harming others is right insofar as it is the refraining from inflicting harm. This is a morally significant way to relate to other persons. Another

---

25. Beauchamp and Childress, *Principles of Biomedical Ethics*, pp. 210-11.
26. W. D. Ross, *The Right and the Good* (Oxford: Clarendon Press, 1930), ch. 2.

morally significant relation is one that individuals have to themselves. Ross identifies duties of self-improvement, those of increasing in virtue or intelligence. In the analysis that follows, I will be seeking to identify morally significant relations that make up right- or wrong-making characteristics of actions. This will identify aspects of comfort-only care, PAS, and euthanasia not noticed or attended to by Beauchamp and Childress.

Let us begin with the example of increasing pain relief near the end of life to a degree that knowingly has a high probability of hastening death. Beauchamp and Childress would claim that engaging in this practice at the request of the terminally ill patient is an act that intends not only to relieve pain but also to end life. If this intentional hastening of death is morally acceptable, it should be equally morally acceptable to hasten death by providing a lethal dose of medication (PAS) or a lethal injection (euthanasia) at the request of a patient who requests it for relief of pain that would otherwise require massive, life-compromising dosages to relieve. Indeed, why not end the pain even more quickly, if that is agreeable to the physician and patient? At first blush these acts appear to share the same moral characteristics: the right-making characteristic of relieving pain; and the wrong-making characteristic of ending a life.

But there are other morally significant aspects of these acts to consider. When physicians assist in a suicide or engage in euthanasia, they introduce into the physician/patient relation a lethal agent. Employing an agent known to be lethal relates the physician to the patient in one of the ways that a murderer relates to the one who is killed, namely injuring them with lethal means. The restraint against using means incompatible with the life of another human being has to be overcome. This directly undermines the usual inhibitions against killing that generally govern in human relations. In using an agent that relieves pain in dosages that are not known to be lethal until a dose becomes the final one, there is still an interaction with the patient as one who continues to live. Respect for the life of the patient persists and in some cases, pain relief even successfully prolongs life and eases pain. In any event, when the patient dies in comfort-only care, death results from the interaction between the condition of the patient and the intervention, not from the intervention alone. Lethal means are the single cause of death in acts of PAS and euthanasia; the weakened condition of the patient is irrelevant to the cause of death. The one using medication to relieve pain is concerned about the condition of the patient as a living individual up to the moment of death. The inhibition against killing is no more adversely affected, if it is at all, than in undertaking high-risk, emergency surgery to save a life, and failing. Furthermore, in the case of a terminally ill patient, you know that the death of the patient is not something you can prevent, but only delay, by providing pain relief in measured amounts rather than amounts known to be immediately lethal. This is respect for life. This is refraining from killing unjustifiably as we usually understand it, that is, refraining from the use of means known to be lethal *in themselves* for the purpose of ending someone's life.

Respect for life also entails the wish that the other individual live. There is no necessity to give up that wish in the absence of engaging in acts by means that are known to kill. As a physician you remain willing to care for your patient; as a patient you remain willing to be cared for. Someone like Quill sees no value in these few extra days or even weeks, living in such dependence on the help of others. He is utterly opposed to laws that do not allow PAS for patients whose pain, in the end, can only be controlled by sedation. Respect for life should be reserved for a life that the patient would deem to be worth living. Beauchamp and Childress also stress what they consider to be the centrality of quality-of-life judgments.[27] They reject the proposal of the ethicist Paul Ramsey to limit judgments about when it is justifiable to refuse life-sustaining treatments to strictly medical indications.[28] For permanently unconscious patients, and that could include patients fully sedated in their last hours or days, they do not regard what they refer to as "mere biological life" to be a benefit. Maintenance of such a life could only be a benefit if the diagnosis or prognosis is wrong, and a medical breakthrough occurs before the individual dies. But Ramsey opposes this shift, from assessing whether treatments are beneficial to patients, to assessing whether patients' lives are beneficial to them. Beauchamp and Childress reject the basis of Ramsey's objection to this shift; namely that it opens the door to involuntary euthanasia. But Ramsey has uncovered a critical element about treatment decisions. Once you begin to ground decisions that may result in hastening death or immediate death on an evaluation of the quality of anyone's life, you have introduced a mode of moral thinking that views some patients as having such a low quality of life if their life continues that it is better for them to die than to receive comfort-only care. That is exactly the justification offered by Dutch physicians who violate the guidelines that permit voluntary euthanasia: they end the lives of some competent patients without their consent because these patients had such a low quality of life at the time and prospectively.[29] Ramsey's point has certainly proved plausible, possibly totally

27. Beauchamp and Childress, *Principles of Biomedical Ethics*, pp. 215-19.
28. Beauchamp and Childress, *Principles of Biomedical Ethics*, pp. 215-16.
29. See, for example, John Keown, "Euthanasia in the Netherlands: Sliding Down the Slippery Slope?" *Notre Dame Journal of Law, Ethics and Public Policy* 9, no. 2 (1995), citing, on page 428, data showing that in 31 percent of 1,000 cases of involuntary euthanasia,

correct, though Beauchamp and Childress, as well as others, remain unpersuaded for reasons I will explore more fully in the next chapter. What occupies us now is that Beauchamp and Childress do not at this juncture give credence to a very important moral element that distinguishes comfort-only treatment from PAS and euthanasia. I refer to the manifestation of respect for life that takes place whenever physicians and patients regard human life as of incalculable worth, and therefore refuse to base their decision on any calculation of its worth. Hence, one reason for choosing sedation rather than PAS or euthanasia is that being sedated for pain relief is like living one's last days sleeping, and living this way does symbolize that the worth of one's life in that condition is not being questioned but respected.

There is another moral reason for choosing sedation, and more generally, comfort-only care rather than PAS or euthanasia. Comfort-only care allows one to sustain the quest to live a virtuous life and even to gain in virtue during one's very last days, weeks, months, or years on earth. With comfort-only care, you can witness to the incalculable worth of human life and the importance of discouraging others from resorting to suicide or euthanasia. By choosing comfort-only care rather than PAS or euthanasia, patients also help retain, in other patients and physicians, the inhibitions against using lethal means to end life directly. These inhibitions certainly have been weakened in Dutch physicians who do not even make the effort to obtain informed consent before deliberately ending the lives of competent patients. Judge Sopinka, writing for the Canadian Supreme Court, explicitly characterized an absolute ban on assisted suicide as an effort to prevent anyone tempted to commit suicide from doing so.[30] In this way Sopinka is portraying one thing he expects from the law, namely an inhibitory effect on behavior that is destructive of human life.

Beauchamp and Childress might find some of these additional morally significant relations interesting, and may even agree that they merit discussion. However, they could argue that they too respect life and they favor safeguards against involuntary euthanasia as well as good-faith efforts to offer alternatives to PAS and euthanasia. But in the last analysis, they claim that the individual who requests a quick painless death, and the physician who complies, should be free, by mutual agreement, to act accordingly. They do not view these actions as in any way morally unjustifiable. No one should or need

physicians gave "low quality of life" as their justification for such acts. See also Henck Jochemsen, "The Netherlands Experiment," in John F. Kilner, Arlene B. Miller, and Edmund D. Pellegrino, eds., *Dignity and Dying: A Christian Appraisal* (Grand Rapids: Eerdmans, 1996).

30. *Rodriguez v. British Columbia,* 107 D.L.R. 4th 342 (1993).

be harmed by PAS or euthanasia under the conditions that justify comfort-only care. The decisions to resort to PAS or euthanasia involve respect for the autonomy of the agents. They do nothing that is inconsistent with virtue. Indeed, respect for autonomy is, for them, a moral principle. Furthermore, Beauchamp and Childress take the view that, if an individual

> desires death rather than life's more typical goods and projects, then causing that person's death at his or her autonomous request does not either harm or wrong the person (though it might still harm others or society by setting back their interests, which might be a reason against the practice).[31]

In their view, the wrong in killing is that the individuals killed are deprived of interests they might otherwise pursue and lose the very capacity to plan and choose a future in pursuit of their interests.[32] But if an individual desires death, Beauchamp and Childress presume that they have no further interests they wish to pursue and so cannot be harmed by taking their lives or having them taken. One could say that for Beauchamp and Childress life has lost all of its worth, at least all worth that may be regarded as morally significant. Add to this account that individuals who see no worth in pursuing life plan to escape from suffering; it is then the case that denying their plans is the harm that should be avoided. So, at least, Beauchamp and Childress contend.

Having identified to their satisfaction what is wrong about killing when it is wrong, Beauchamp and Childress return to the central concern discussed in this chapter when they conclude that

> those who believe it is sometimes morally acceptable to let people die but not to take active steps to help them die must therefore give a different account of the wrongfulness of killing persons than the one we have suggested. The burden of justification, then, seems to rest on those who would refuse assistance to those who wish to die, rather than on those who would help them.[33]

Beauchamp and Childress are certainly right that those who morally justify some instances of comfort-only care but no instances of PAS and euthanasia must give "a different account of the wrongfulness of killing" than the one they suggest. Indeed, that is precisely what I will be doing in Chapter Three. But in claiming that those who find PAS and euthanasia morally unjustifiable have the burden of proof, they are begging the question about

31. Beauchamp and Childress, *Principles of Biomedical Ethics*, p. 236.
32. Beauchamp and Childress, *Principles of Biomedical Ethics*, p. 236.
33. Beauchamp and Childress, *Principles of Biomedical Ethics*, p. 236.

whether comfort-only care differs morally from PAS and euthanasia. In the end, their failure to find a moral difference between comfort-only care and PAS and euthanasia rests on their particular claims as to what makes killing wrong when it is wrong. They find nothing morally wrong about giving approval to a request for lethal means to end life from those who can find no reason for continuing to live. In Chapter Three I will discuss why this view, if adopted, provides no principled reason for preventing anyone who despairs of life or finds life meaningless, from committing suicide. Indeed, as I will argue, Beauchamp and Childress have abandoned, or at least undermined, the moral structure that serves as the principled basis for homicide law.

CHAPTER THREE

The Moral Structure of
Life's Worth and Protection

This book began with a consideration of suffering. Although it is clear from that first chapter on suffering that there are excellent alternatives to PAS as a response to suffering; and, although it is clear also that comfort-only care can suppress the desire for PAS, those who advocate PAS and its legalization tend to be unpersuaded by the data, however impressive. One reason given is that comfort-only care that hastens death is legally permitted, so why not permit PAS, or also euthanasia, since it secures the very same end? And so Chapter Two suggested some ways in which comfort-only care, when it is morally justified, differs from PAS. But the case for such differences needs to be considerably extended. As noted in the preceding chapter, Beauchamp and Childress based their view, for morally equating comfort care that hastens death with PAS and euthanasia, on their particular account of what is wrong with causing death when it is wrong. In this chapter, I will reject that view: I will depict and defend an alternative view of the moral structure, a structure that upholds life's worth, and that presently serves as the moral basis for homicide law and the legal bans of assisted suicide and euthanasia.

The Wrongness of Killing: The Moral Requisites
of Individual and Communal Life

As noted above, Beauchamp and Childress find no significant moral difference between comfort-only care that hastens death and PAS and euthanasia, given the same circumstances in which dying patients are now legally permitted to request and receive comfort-only care. They argue that

45

What makes it [causing death] wrong, when it is wrong, is that a person is harmed — that is, suffers a setback to interests that the person otherwise would not have experienced. In particular one is caused the loss of the capacity to plan and choose a future, together with a deprivation of expectable goods. This explains why inflicting death both harms and wrongs a person.[1]

From this line of reasoning, Beauchamp and Childress conclude that for an individual who "desires death rather than life's more typical goods and projects . . . causing that person's death at his or her autonomous request does not either harm or wrong the person. . . ."[2] Whether one arranges for death by refusing life-sustaining treatment or requesting PAS, the fact that death is willed, that is, knowingly chosen, means that those who in either instance cause death have harmed no one. For Beauchamp and Childress, PAS and active, voluntary euthanasia do not differ in this regard. The key ingredient that justifies arranging for one's death, whether by refusing life-sustaining treatment, or requesting PAS or euthanasia, is that the one whose death it is freely requests the arrangement and hence is not harmed.

Given this view of the harmlessness of requesting death, Beauchamp and Childress argue that patients in very burdensome circumstances are harmed if PAS is not legally permitted and no one honors their requests to have their lives ended. Since patients who will very soon die when life-sustaining treatment is withdrawn or not initiated do have their right to autonomy honored, the failure to grant the same right to lingering patients in equally unbearable circumstances "seems tantamount to condemning the patient to a life he or she does not want."[3]

There are two things Beauchamp and Childress say individuals stand to lose when they lose their lives: (1) the capacity to plan and choose a future; (2) life's more typical goods and projects. These losses are the harms that make killing wrong when it is wrong. But, on this view, if individuals no longer want the capacity to plan and choose a future, the loss of this capacity is not a harm. And, if individuals do not want any more of the goods expected from continuing to live, the loss of them is also not a harm. Notice that Beauchamp and Childress do not posit life itself as a good, and certainly not as an inalienable right. Rather, life is a right only if individuals desire and claim it; life is good only as a means to whatever individuals regard as good.

---

1. Tom L. Beauchamp and James F. Childress, *Principles of Biomedical Ethics*, 4th ed. (New York: Oxford University Press, 1994), p. 236.

2. Beauchamp and Childress, *Principles of Biomedical Ethics*, p. 236.

3. Beauchamp and Childress, *Principles of Biomedical Ethics*, p. 226.

Now Beauchamp and Childress might desire to interrupt the discussion at this point to remind us that the context in which they are speaking about individuals as being condemned to lives they may not wish to live is one of dying under very undesirable, even intolerable, circumstances. Even so, it is fair to ask whether it is the perspective of such dying individuals that is to prevail or that of others. If, as Beauchamp and Childress claim, autonomy is the key reason for granting individuals legal permission to request PAS and euthanasia, then it should be the perceptions of those who regard their own lives as intolerable that should prevail in granting such requests. Beauchamp and Childress do not provide a reason to say to such individuals, given that they are competent, "You ought to desire to live when you are not terminally ill, not in physical pain, and not in anyway debilitated or incapacitated." They could presume that, absent any of these maladies, people would not commit suicide or seek death. But they undoubtedly do not so presume since people do commit suicide under a variety of circumstances. It is more likely Beauchamp and Childress are trying to carve out a special, private sphere within which autonomy reigns, a sphere comparable to those whose death can be hastened by comfort-only care when they are terminally ill and near death. However, they do so without offering a principled reason for preventing suicides. In principle, the only reason they give for preventing suicide or euthanasia is that people should not be killed, or assisted in killing themselves, when they express no wish to have this happen. Beauchamp and Childress do not offer us a reason why, under some circumstances at least, individuals ought to have no desire to kill themselves or be killed.

Since Beauchamp and Childress consider it harmful, morally and legally, to fail to grant a dying patient's request for PAS, and since they provide no principled reason to prevent suicide when it is desired, they leave hospice care without any clear moral justification. Hospice was founded to provide comfort-only care that would help prevent suicide and euthanasia. Hospice physicians repeatedly report that once they provide comfort-only care, patients who expressed a desire to end their lives, or have it ended, change their minds, or else no longer pursue ending their lives as an option.[4] Strictly speaking, Beauchamp and Childress have posited situations in which attempts to change a patient's openly expressed wish for an immediate end to the dying process are morally wrong, even reprehensible. At the same time,

---

4. See, for example, Robert G. Twycross, "Where There Is Hope, There Is Life: A View from the Hospice," in John Keown, ed., *Euthanasia Examined: Ethical, Clinical and Legal Perspectives* (Cambridge: Cambridge University Press, 1995), pp. 141-68. See the many cases, studies, and publications cited by Twycross.

the situations they treat as unchangeable, or as ones that should not be changed, cannot and will not be changed unless the attempt is made to change those situations, as hospice does so successfully.

The question before us, then, remains: Is there any moral justification for providing comfort-only care rather than PAS or euthanasia in conditions that patients, at the time, regard as hopelessly undesirable, and in the light of which patients ask to have their lives ended? The answer to this question requires an account of why PAS and euthanasia cannot be morally justified. To make this case, it is necessary to say what moral structures and responsibilities are violated by the decisions and actions these practices entail.

On June 26, 1997, the United States Supreme Court announced its unanimous decisions to uphold the constitutionality of the laws totally prohibiting assisted suicide in the states of Washington and New York.[5] Writing for the Supreme Court, Chief Justice Rehnquist ruled that there is no constitutionally protected "right to commit suicide which itself includes a right to assistance in doing so." He found that "for over 700 years Anglo-American common law tradition has punished or otherwise disapproved of both suicide and assisting suicide."[6] This tradition continues to be reflected in law.[7] Indeed, an analysis of Chief Justice Rehnquist's reference to this tradition, embedded in current as well as past law, revealed that there are at least three major reasons that killing is wrong when it is wrong: (1) killing is a violation of an individual's inalienable right to life; (2) killing runs counter to a human being's natural love of life; and (3) killing violates the sanctity of life. Now I wish to identify the moral structure that provides a moral justification for these reasons for the wrongfulness of killing. As I do so, I will show as well why this moral structure provides a reasonable justification for the laws forbidding assistance in a suicide, and for homicide law as such.

The Natural Inalienable Right to Life

Rather than begin with a definition of "natural" and "inalienable," I will allow their meaning to emerge as the case for describing the right to life in these ways is being developed. In the legal reasoning cited by Chief Justice Rehnquist, the right to life is also described as "sacred." I will take up what it means to call life sacred below in the section devoted to an extensive discussion of life's sacred-

5. *Washington v. Glucksberg,* 117 S.Ct. 2258 (1997); *Vacco v. Quill,* 117 S.Ct. 2293 (1997).
6. *Washington v. Glucksberg,* 2263.
7. *Washington v. Glucksberg,* 2263.

ness, as understood in law and in morality, and the moral justification for its evocation as a standard for guiding legal and moral practices.

As indicated in Chapter One, the contemporary moral philosopher Alan Gewirth has mounted a strong defense of natural human rights.[8] He locates morality within the domain of human actions. Seeking to base the claims that moral rights make upon our actions, on reason, and not upon utility or contingent desires or attitudes, he asks what conditions are logically necessary if human agents are to achieve by their actions any of their purposes whatsoever. He identifies freedom and well-being, including life, as the procedural and substantive conditions necessary to pursue and achieve the goods agents seek. Freedom and well-being, life included, are the objects of rights, that is, what one has a right to. Rights are moral, for Gewirth, because they are justifiable through a valid moral principle; a principle is "moral" in that it identifies the categorically obligatory nature of certain requirements of action. These requirements are equally requirements for all actual or prospective agents, and serve important interests all agents or recipients equally share.

But Gewirth has not completely and consistently followed his own method of explicating the logically necessary, universal conditions for human agency. He takes autonomous individuals as his starting point. What Gewirth has not considered are the conditions necessary logically and functionally for there to be individual human beings and agents at all. He portrays human beings as agents without regard to the fact that they cease and come to be: Individual human agents can neither come to be nor persist on their own. Human beings only exist and act because of the cooperative behavior of other human agents.

To begin with, human beings come to be and persist through procreation, nurture, instruction, and a whole array of actions, practices, and agencies that protect human life and well-being. There are, then, certain proclivities that make a human life possible at all: the proclivities to procreate and nurture. There are other proclivities essential to the continuation of a human life: the proclivities to nurture and protect life. Then there are as well certain inhibitions essential to the continuation of a human life: there are the inhibitions against killing, against taking away, or failing to provide, the necessities of life, and against lying. It should be noted that lying as a practice can undermine the whole network — social, legal, and educational — that protects human life. All of these proclivities and inhibitions, and the individual and communal behavior they make possible, also are requisite for the realization

8. Alan Gewirth, *Reason and Morality* (Chicago: University of Chicago Press, 1978), and *Human Rights: Essays on Justification and Applications* (Chicago: University of Chicago Press, 1982).

and sustenance of human freedom. The individual freedom to pursue one's purposes can be undermined or thwarted by a lack of nurture and instruction, or by lying, stealing, or ultimately, by being killed or killing oneself.

Human rights, then, cannot simply be rendered actual by claiming them, or by asserting or proving their necessity for achieving our individual purposes. Human rights only become actual through actions, patterns of behavior, and social arrangements that render their actualization possible. I came to be by the loving procreative, nurturant, and life-protecting behavior of my parents and the social and legal entities in the community in which my parents lived. My life persisted because the proclivities and inhibitions protecting life persisted in the behavior of my parents and members of my larger community.[9] For these reasons, or reasons like these, my life and the lives of all other individual human beings now persist. For these reasons, or reasons like these, communities came to be and exist. No community can come to be, or continue to exist, without some procreation and nurture of human life, and without behavior that is sufficiently restrained by the inhibitions against killing, lying, and stealing. These behaviors and behavioral constraints constitute morally significant relations between and among individuals and groups.[10] What, then, does it mean to assert that human rights become actual through the behavior patterns that create and sustain these morally significant relations, behavior patterns I will henceforth call morally responsible?

To begin with, behaving in these morally responsible ways is exhibited by and expected from individuals and communities. These behaviors are "natural" both in the sense of being actual or real, and in the sense of being a continuous, predictable set of occurrences: they evoke expectations. Having brought a child into being, and nurtured, educated, and protected it, parents expect, even seek similar proclivities and inhibitions in that child. In turn, other members of any larger community expect that parents will be morally responsible, that is, provide for the nurture, education, and necessities of life for the child they spawned. Indeed, their expectations are such that it is ap-

9. As I am using the term "community," families as well as nations and their subdivisions can qualify as communities: "A community is *an affiliated and mutually beneficial network of interdependent beings who, as human beings, share what is requisite for forming and sustaining such a network.*" Arthur J. Dyck, *Rethinking Rights and Responsibilities: The Moral Bonds of Community* (Cleveland: Pilgrim Press, 1994), p. 126. Each key term in this definition is explained on pages 126 and 127.

10. Another morally significant relation, a requisite of familial life and the nurture of children, is sexual fidelity within the marital relation. The use of the term "moral" is something I have discussed extensively in my book, *Rethinking Rights and Responsibilities*, cited above, in chapters 7-9.

propriate to say that the child has a right to the necessities of life and to life itself. Should the parents fail to meet these expectations by threatening the right of their child to life, that right will become a right claimed on behalf of that child by the community through its legally authorized agencies to try to assure that the right is not violated. Parents may even lose custody of that child so that others will be free to meet the moral responsibilities owed the child, and thereby prevent the violation of its rights. Needless to say, irresponsible behavior that results in death is subject to legal punishments for anyone who violated that child's right to life.

Rights, then, exist continuously and naturally as expectations that our natural moral responsibilities, requisite to individual and communal life, will be met. Given the continuity of these requisites, we are not usually any more conscious of these expectations than we are of the continuity of the law of gravity that also is a requisite of our activities on earth. But, when any of these moral responsibilities are not met, our expectations tend to turn into claims on behalf of the individuals or groups who are threatened by such failures of what we otherwise expect as a matter of course. Human rights, then, can be said to be actual, either as expectations or claims on the human relations that are moral requisites of our individual and communal life.

Human rights are inalienable. They are rendered actual as expectations of, or claims upon, a continuous set of morally significant human relations, created by natural proclivities and inhibitions that also sustain these relations. Consider the simple fact that each of us is the offspring of parents. We owe them our lives. We also owe our lives to the larger community in which their behavior and our lives were undergirded and protected. What we owe was made possible by the morally responsible behavior I have identified as the moral requisites of individual and communal life. In turn, all of those who have sustained our lives, and still do, expect from us and stand ready to claim from us, behavior that is in accord with these same moral requisites of individual and communal life. We cannot, by wishing it to be so, divest ourselves, or anyone else, of these responsibilities and the rights they render actual. They belong to all of us as individuals and members of communities. They are inalienable.

Now consider what is implied by this account of the inalienability of the right to life. Ronald Dworkin and five other moral philosophers submitted an Amicus Curiae Brief to the Supreme Court in support of an individual right to PAS.[11] In this brief, they recognized that the state has interests that would

---

11. Ronald Dworkin, Thomas Nagel, Robert Nozick, John Rawls, Thomas Scanlon, and Judith Jarvis Thomson had this brief published as "Assisted Suicide: The Philosophers'

justify denying some requests for PAS. The state could do so out of concern
for those people who are not terminally ill but who have nevertheless formed
a desire to die. The reason the state could legitimate denying PAS to this
group of persons is that they "are, as a group, very likely later to be grateful if
they are prevented from taking their own lives."[12] These authors are making
gratitude for one's life contingent upon whether or not people actually feel it.
This is not surprising given the fact that their basis for favoring a right to PAS
is that the Supreme Court should recognize that an individual has a right to
live or die on the basis of "his own convictions about why his life is valuable
and where its value lies."[13] Dworkin et alia have provided us no basis for saying that each of us *ought* to be grateful for our lives. Our lives did not and
could not originate and persist because we valued it but because someone else
valued it, parents to begin with, but also a whole network of individuals and
groups. Our lives depended upon and continue to depend on the persistence
of the moral behavior that makes life, and the communal protection of it,
possible at all. This behavior is expected and claimed as a right by all. What
we owe, then, is to behave in these same ways. Whether in living in accord
with the moral responsibilities that initiate and sustain individuals and communal life we feel gratitude or not, we are doing what a grateful individual
would do, namely doing unto others as they have done unto us. This we
ought to do. And to do it out of gratitude would be virtuous and would
strengthen the proclivities and inhibitions to act as we ought. What we owe
one another are responsibilities that remain, whether we live up to them or
not. They are the inalienable natural bases of our rights. Being terminally ill
does not change this reality.

But, is it not the case that, despite the continuities exhibited by the proclivities and inhibitions that actualize the moral requisites of individual and
communal life, individuals and groups violate or break with these continuously binding moral responsibilities humans have toward one another? There
is no question that individuals and groups sometimes act in ways that run
counter to their moral responsibilities.[14] That is why it is universally deemed

Brief," in *The New York Review*, March 27, 1997, pp. 41-47. Hereafter, page references to this
brief will be to its fully reprinted locus in *Issues in Law and Medicine* 15, no. 2 (Fall 1997):
183-98 and identified as "Brief of Ronald Dworkin et al."

12. "Brief of Ronald Dworkin et al.," p. 196.

13. "Brief of Ronald Dworkin et al.," p. 197.

14. Someone like Reinhold Niebuhr would state the matter much more strongly: All
of our actions less than fully meet our moral responsibilities. Indeed, in *Moral Man and
Immoral Society* (New York: Charles Scribner's Sons, 1932), Niebuhr argued that actions
carried out by groups, and on behalf of groups, were always tainted by the biases and loyal-

necessary to have laws, law enforcement agencies, and military forces, in order to try to prevent killing and even threats to assault or kill human beings. Were I deliberately to kill an innocent person, that is, kill an individual who is not threatening my life in any way, I would be breaking with the shared mutual responsibilities to protect human life. In doing this, I would have overcome my inhibitions against killing in such a way that I would be rightly seen as a threat to all other human beings. I would also correctly be seen as a threat to the inhibitions against killing present in my larger community, particularly those of individuals, families, or other groups who had great affection for the victim. In short, I would have become a threat to others and to the moral fabric of my community. To deal with this, my larger community would try to neutralize and ward off these threats by depriving me of my usual rights to freedom.[15] Apart from exceptions such as unavoidable accidents and self-defense, killing individuals evokes responses, through laws and enforcement agencies, that attempt to neutralize or otherwise remove any threat to others and to the moral requisites of individual and communal life that any individual or group may pose, were they to kill and remain free and unpunished.

What about killing oneself? In this instance as well the moral responsibilities to protect human life are violated and the inhibitions of others against killing are threatened. Indeed, we know as a matter of fact that there are copycat suicides as well as murders. Highly publicized suicides are almost invariably followed by other suicides. The moral responsibility to prevent the death of individuals, innocent of any crime, is, as noted above, continuous. Committing suicide is a failure in such a moral responsibility. The policy in place in the United States does not call for punishing anyone in the event of an unassisted suicide. That is justifiable. For one thing, any punishment of the victim would adversely affect only those who had close ties with that individual and, if they did not assist in or encourage that individual to commit suicide, they in no way, relative to this event, have done anything to threaten others or the moral fabric. Second, it is always possible that the individual committing suicide cannot be held morally responsible for what they did because they were clinically depressed. There is no fair way to judge that. However, those who advocate PAS are urging that suicide can be rational, and hence those who commit it can be held morally responsible for what they do. Those who see themselves as rationally and intentionally justified in killing themselves are intending to act

---

ties of those belonging to the groups in question. Thus Niebuhr was quick to call attention to the evils that, for him, made World War II necessary and to the evils perpetrated by all the nations participating in that war.

15. The punishments for killing vary, of course, from imprisonment to capital punishment within nations and among the nations.

in a way that violates and threatens our mutual moral responsibilities to one another. Furthermore, they are encouraging such actions.

What about those who willingly assist in a suicide? They are willing accomplices in behavior that violates and threatens the moral fabric of our communities in the ways depicted above. What is more, their willingness to assist is an encouragement to someone seriously contemplating suicide. At the time of a study of hospice patients in England, none of the patients who had AIDS and asked to have their lives ended actually persisted in their requests.[16] In the Netherlands, under the care of physicians willing to assist AIDS patients to end their lives, and legally permitted to do so, euthanasia was administered in 30 percent of the cases.[17] What happens in the Netherlands illustrates both the influence of physicians on patients, and the influence of laws on both. Law does have a pedagogical effect on behavior.[18] Furthermore, the inhibitions of medical professionals against killing have been weakened in the Netherlands. Witness the documented instances of involuntary euthanasia and the reasons given for carrying them out, despite the legal criteria forbidding euthanasia without informed consent.[19]

Killing, then, is wrong when the act of killing oneself or someone else violates and threatens to undermine the mutual moral responsibilities that are requisites of individual and communal life. In so doing they violate that individual's natural and inalienable right to life, and all the expectations and claims it makes on human behavior.

But killing can be wrong also when it is an act that no longer exhibits a love for life. The moral structure depicted above is not recognized as such by those who do not judge what is moral from the standpoint of wishing the self and the other to exist. What is the role of "love of life" in morality? That is the question we will now address.

16. Reported in Robert G. Twycross, "Where There Is Hope, There Is Life," pp. 152-54.

17. Twycross, "Where There Is Hope, There Is Life," pp. 152-54.

18. Mary Ann Glendon discusses the law as a teacher in *Rights Talk: The Impoverishment of Political Discourse* (New York: Free Press, 1991), pp. 85-88, including a study of how law guides one's conduct and opinions.

19. See Carlos Gomez, *Regulating Death: Euthanasia and the Case of the Netherlands* (New York: Free Press, 1991); Herbert Hendin, *Seduced by Death: Doctors, Patients and the Dutch Cure* (New York: W. W. Norton, 1997). Hendin's work has many further references. See also p. 11, n. 2.

The Love of Life

The affirmation that human beings love life is found in law. The love of life was evoked by the U.S. Supreme Court. Writing for the Court, Chief Justice Rehnquist cited Zephaniah Swift, a legal theorist who became Chief Justice of Connecticut. Having argued the case for abolishing punishment for suicide, Swift indicated why he thought that such a change in the law would not be harmful to society. Suicide, he wrote, "is so abhorrent to the feelings of mankind, and that strong love of life which is implanted in the human heart, that it cannot be so frequently committed, as to become dangerous to society."[20] Rehnquist took Swift's statement as a clear indication that the unwillingness to punish suicide did not constitute an acceptance of suicide. Subsequent court opinions, and Rehnquist provided some examples, did indeed repudiate suicide as commendable and as a right.[21]

What is the moral significance of viewing killing oneself, and killing as such, as acts that are contrary to, and in violation of, the love of life that is implanted in us and naturally characteristic of us as human beings? One implication of taking the view that human beings naturally love life is to consider those who lose the love for their lives as deviating from normal behavior and disturbed in some way.[22] According to one source, 95 percent of those who commit suicide had a major psychiatric illness at the time of death.[23] Furthermore, experiencing pain can lead to depression, and those who are treated for depression and relieved of pain are then "grateful to be alive."[24] From a moral standpoint, attributing mental stress or illness to those who commit suicide alleviates them of any moral responsibility for killing themselves; they were not rational when they committed suicide. Accordingly, the loss of love for one's life is something that individuals and societies should always seek to correct; to do so successfully is to remove some sources of emotional or mental distress.

But apart from the extent to which the loss of love for one's life may or may not be associated with mental illness, losing love for one's life does impair moral cognition. Aristotle identified this relationship between loving one's own life and moral knowledge in his account of what it means to be a

---

20. *Washington v. Glucksberg,* 2264.

21. *Washington v. Glucksberg,* 2264.

22. The psychiatrist Peter Sainsbury is among those mental health experts who take the view that all individuals who express a wish to commit suicide are in need of medical intervention. See his chapter, "Community Psychiatry," in Seymour Perlin, ed., *A Handbook for the Study of Suicide* (New York: Oxford University Press, 1975), pp. 165-84.

23. *Washington v. Glucksberg,* 2272.

24. *Washington v. Glucksberg,* 2272-73.

friend. To begin with, he noted that friendly relations between neighbors as well as the defining characteristics of friendships are known and attainable because of the relationships individuals have to themselves. The good we wish and do for ourselves is what we wish and do for our friends. One of the good things we wish for ourselves is to exist and live. That wish is one of the qualities that defines what it means to be a friend: "one who wishes his friend to exist and live, for his sake; which mothers do to their children."[25] This relationship of wishing oneself and another to live is a form of love, for as Aristotle says of love, it is "ideally an excess of friendship."[26] Those who love their own lives, then, know how to behave towards a neighbor and a friend; they know what it is to be a friend.

By invoking the love of mothers for their children, Aristotle is equating the love individuals have for their own lives with the natural proclivities that fuel procreation, nurture, and the wishes parents have that their children live and more.[27] Love for oneself and others, expressed in wishing oneself and others to exist, is, then, for Aristotle a natural expression of love, like that of being a parent. However, these natural expressions of love can be weakened or undermined. One source for this, as Aristotle describes it, is that people can be at variance with themselves as they follow their own desires:

> This is true, for instance, of incontinent people; for they choose instead of the things they themselves think good, things that are pleasant but hurtful; while others again, through cowardice and laziness, shrink from doing what they think best for themselves.[28]

And individuals "who have done many terrible deeds and are hated for their wickedness even shrink from life and destroy themselves."[29] So, for Aristotle, the diminution or extinction of the love of one's life is not only possible, but may even result in the destruction of one's own life. For as Aristotle observes of wicked people that, "having nothing loveable in them, they have no feeling of love to themselves."[30] Such individuals, then, lack the attributes needed to

---

25. Aristotle, *Nichomachean Ethics,* Book IX, Ch. 4.

26. Aristotle, *Nichomachean Ethics,* Book IX, Ch. 10.

27. In a transcultural study, the psychologist Tamara Dembo found that parents and future parents wish "health," "economic security," "knowledge" or "intelligence," and "happy marriage" (or "loving" or "being loved"). Reported in Charles Reynolds, "Elements of a Decision Procedure for Christian Social Ethics," *Harvard Theological Review* 65, no. 4 (October 1972): 513-14.

28. Aristotle, *Nichomachean Ethics,* Book IX, Ch. 4.

29. Aristotle, *Nichomachean Ethics,* Book IX, Ch. 4.

30. Aristotle, *Nichomachean Ethics,* Book IX, Ch. 4.

know how to be a friend or be moved to be one; they will also lack the attributes characteristic of parental love and the understanding of what it takes to be a loving parent.

The diminution or loss of love for oneself and for one's life distorts moral cognition. Our knowledge of how we ought to behave towards others is very much dependent on knowing what is morally right behavior toward ourselves: It is wrong for you to kill or try to kill me, and hence I have a basis for thinking it would be wrong to kill or try to kill you. But if I do not wish myself to exist I may not perceive the fact that others *do* wish to live. Not wishing to exist, I may not regard it as wrong to be killed or to kill myself. But then I may also not regard it as wrong to kill you or to assist you to kill yourself. Since I do not wish myself to exist, I may well assume that you also do not wish to exist, even if you do not express such a wish. Furthermore, I may tend to misperceive the wishes of those who do say they do not wish to live. They may be speaking out of their pain or mental distress, or they may be seeking affirmation of their lives as worthy of existence, but in the absence of a wish that I exist, I may not recognize the wish to exist in others. Indeed, I may even think that people who wish to live under certain circumstances are irrational; lacking a wish that I exist, I do not expect others to wish to live in circumstances that I regard as worse than anything I am experiencing.

Someone might object to this line of reasoning. What would be wrong, they might contend, with wishing myself to exist but imagining that I and anyone else might understandably lose that wish under very dire circumstances when dying and near death? One can grant that such a loss of the wish to live is not only understandable but does indeed occur, though temporarily, for the great majority who are successfully treated for pain and/or clinical depression, a point discussed and documented previously. However, as I argued in the section above, our inalienable right to life rests upon our continuous and natural moral responsibilities to nurture and protect our lives. The wish no longer to assume this responsibility is a failure, either in our willingness or our emotional or mental capacity to meet that responsibility. The argument I am now putting forward is that the failure to meet that moral responsibility, whether intentionally or in circumstances beyond our control, distorts our perceptions of reality, and hence also our ability to know what is right. For those who are dying, such cognitive distortions can be corrected. Obviously such changes from wishing to die to wishing to live, as the perspective from which to make moral decisions, can only occur if the efforts to bring about such changes are seen as right and are actually undertaken.

Aristotle, as quoted above, observed that people who have done many evil things will find nothing lovable in themselves and hence will not have feelings of love toward themselves. But this phenomenon obtains not only for those who have a history of doing evil, but tragically it occurs also for those who are dying, particularly those in a state of great or even complete dependence upon care from others. Individuals, highly or completely dependent on others, can come to view themselves as not at all lovable anymore. Indeed, the question of how one will be remembered, whether as vibrant, active, and attractive or as relatively helpless, debilitated, and unattractive, are among the reasons some give for wishing to end one's life either to ward off or cut short a progressive process of physical and/or mental deterioration.[31] In addition, then, to the best of care in treating pain, depression, and fear of death, it is important to address what purpose is served by dying persons who do not request PAS or euthanasia. Simply stated, such individuals fulfill some very important moral responsibilities. First of all, they do not repudiate the worth of their lives or anyone else's. Second, they show no ingratitude to those who brought them into being and nurtured them, those who help protect their lives, and those who have so far sustained their lives through all of their illnesses. Third, they encourage no one to overcome their inhibitions against killing themselves, assisting others to do so, or killing others. Fourth, they directly encourage those who are experiencing illnesses that may only temporarily or partially render them quite helpless, or disfigured, or dependent on others, to persist in that state and sustain their hope that the love for their lives will be sustained and may grow. Fifth, as studies have shown, they create opportunities for spiritual growth, the deepening of existing relationships, and, in some cases, the healing of ruptured relations whether with other persons or the Divine.

These same moral responsibilities and spiritual opportunities that characterize patients who do not request PAS or euthanasia also characterize physicians who do not practice PAS and euthanasia. These patients and physicians help sustain the moral requisites of individual and communal life, and the natural proclivities and inhibitions that structure and uphold our common moral life in this way. By refraining from participation in PAS and euthanasia, physicians and patients, and other potential participants, are also refusing to violate the sacredness of human life.

The Sacredness of Human Life

The idea that life is sacred, like the notion that we naturally love life, has become embedded in law. In 1980, the American Bar Association drew up a

---

31. See *Compassion in Dying v. State of Washington*, 79 F. 3rd 790 (9th Cir. 1996), 814.

Model Penal Code. That Code asserted that "the interests in the sanctity of life are represented in the criminal homicide laws" and are "threatened" by anyone "who expresses a willingness to participate in taking the life of another, even though the act may be accomplished with the consent, or at the request, of the suicide victim."[32] That an individual's life is sacred is continuous and in no way contingent upon life's circumstances: the right to life is both "inalienable" and "sacred."[33] These affirmations are explicitly found in court decisions. The sacredness of life, then, is a key standard found in homicide law for judging the wrongness of killing and assisting in a suicide. How is this standard to be understood, and what justifies its use, morally and legally?

As a standard for judging behavior, sacredness of life is a particular way of characterizing the worth of human life. That a human life is sacred means that the worth of it is beyond calculation, that is, incalculable. One can glean this from what is said about the sanctity of life in law. An individual's life is to be protected in every imaginable circumstance: as a prisoner on death row; as hopelessly ill or fatally wounded; and as one for whom life has in various ways become a burden.[34] In other words, the law's interest in preserving life is unqualified. This interest is not diminished in any way by the medical condition and the wishes of the one whose life is at stake.[35]

As embodied in law, the sacredness of life refers to the incalculable worth of life. In the German Constitutional Court, the judges recognized the necessity of embedding in law the incalculable worth of individual human life. The Weimar Constitution of 1919 had made no explicit reference to the right to life. Mindful of all that had happened during the period of the Nazi regime, the Basic Law of what was then West Germany in 1949 incorporated "the self-evident right to life" and did so "principally as a reaction to the de-

32. *Washington v. Glucksberg,* 2265.

33. *Washington v. Glucksberg,* 2265.

34. *Washington v. Glucksberg,* 2265. The philosopher Francis M. Kamm argues that there are circumstances in which "death is the lesser evil" relative to continuing to live. "Physician-Assisted Suicide, Euthanasia, and Intending Death," in Margaret P. Battin, Rosamond Rhodes, and Anita Silvers, eds., *Physician-Assisted Suicide: Expanding the Debate* (New York: Routledge, 1998), pp. 28-62. This argument, if accepted, would remove the current protection of life that is not contingent upon any of the circumstances Kamm suggests; Kamm does not consider what principle guides, or even should guide, homicide law; she also does not consider how acts of suicide, assisting in them, and euthanasia affect the inhibitions and proclivities essential to the moral requisites of individual and communal life, and essential for effectively enforcing homicide law. She has totally individualized the calculus as to whether it is best to die rather than live with virtually no regard to the ways in which individuals are related to one another.

35. *Washington v. Glucksberg,* 2272.

struction of life unworthy of life."[36] Dr. Benda, writing for the court, made this same point in yet another way. Speaking of the Basic Law, he asserted that

> at its basis lies the concept . . . that human beings possess an inherent worth as individuals in order of creation which uncompromisingly demands unconditional respect for the life of every individual human being, even for the apparently socially "worthless." . . .[37]

What can make killing morally wrong, then, is that a human life, the one killed, is treated as living a life that has little or no worth, rather than as one living a life of incalculable worth and as having a right to be treated accordingly. If laws were permitted to embody the idea that in some circumstances life loses its worth, or that some people lack sufficient worth to have their lives protected, individuals would no longer enjoy equal protection of the law so far as their lives are concerned. Furthermore, some principled basis for protecting human life other than its sanctity would have to be provided to justify what would constitute violations of the unquestioned worth of every individual human life.

Ronald Dworkin has proposed legalizing PAS and also euthanasia because, in doing so, the law would recognize the sacredness of individual human life, not violate it. The basis for his argument is that whether or not the sacredness of life requires death due to natural causes, or death at a time of one's choosing, is a matter of religious belief. People have different beliefs about how their lives should end and what their choices mean. The law should be neutral with regard to these beliefs and should not suppress individual religious beliefs, particularly in such a personal and important matter about which beliefs differ. He makes this point rather strongly when he states that "making someone die in a way that others approve," but the individual whose life it is, "believes" to be "a horrifying contradiction of his life, is a devastating, odious form of tyranny."[38] In what sense, then, is human life sacred for Dworkin? "Something is sacred or inviolable," Dworkin tells us, "when its deliberate destruction would dishonor what ought to be honored."[39]

36. This decision of the West German Federal Constitutional Court is published in full as "West German Abortion Decision: A Contrast to Roe v. Wade?" Robert E. Jonas and John D. Gorby, trans., *John Marshall Journal of Practice and Procedure* 9 (Spring 1976): 605-84. Page references to this decision are to the reprint in S. J. Reiser, A. J. Dyck, and W. J. Curran, eds., *Ethics in Medicine* (Cambridge, Mass.: MIT Press, 1977), p. 417.

37. "West German Abortion Decision," p. 424.

38. Ronald Dworkin, *Life's Dominion: An Argument about Abortion, Euthanasia, and Individual Freedom* (New York: Vintage Books, 1994), p. 217.

39. Dworkin, *Life's Dominion*, p. 74.

Dworkin uses the terms "sacred" and "inviolable" as synonyms. By this definition, how could the deliberate ending of a human life be compatible with its sacredness? Dworkin develops the notion that each individual life represents a whole way of life. Our lives tell a story about us, and how that story ends is very important to us, like the final scene in a drama. For most people, Dworkin contends, how they die has "special, symbolic importance: they want their deaths, if possible to express and in that way vividly to confirm the values they believe most important in their lives."[40] Timing has this kind of significance for "the idea of a good (or less bad) death."[41] In short, Dworkin claims that, "None of us wants to end our lives out of character."[42] For some, dying at the time and in the manner that they choose is the way to respect the inviolability of human life.[43] People's lives differ, and so do their beliefs as to how their own lives should end. Each person's belief about what it will mean to treat their own life as sacred is a personal belief. Dworkin regards that belief as a religious belief. The law should not suppress such religious beliefs because, to do so, violates the sacredness of life as some individuals understand its meaning. These are individuals who believe it is intolerable, utterly undignified, to live under some circumstances that severely limit their physical or mental abilities. Dworkin summarizes his views as follows:

> Because we cherish dignity, we insist on freedom, and we place the right of conscience at its center, so that a government that denies that right is totalitarian no matter how free it leaves us in choices that matter less. Because we have dignity, we demand democracy, and we define it so that a constitution that permits a majority to deny freedom of conscience is democracy's enemy, not its author. Whatever view we take about . . . euthanasia, we want the right to decide for ourselves, and we should therefore be ready to insist that any honorable constitution, any genuine constitution of principle, will guarantee that right for everyone.[44]

In this passage, Dworkin equates a total ban on euthanasia with a totalitarian denial of freedom of conscience. But he is begging the question. The question is about practices that should or should not be permitted by law. First I would distinguish between a religious belief and the actions or prac-

---

40. Dworkin, *Life's Dominion*, p. 211. This concern with what one's death expresses is also about how one is remembered (p. 210).

41. Dworkin, *Life's Dominion*, p. 211.

42. Dworkin, *Life's Dominion*, p. 213.

43. Dworkin, *Life's Dominion*, p. 216.

44. Dworkin, *Life's Dominion*, p. 239.

tices favored by that belief. There have been, and still are, people whose religious beliefs incline them to favor polygamy. However, the Supreme Court and the laws of the land do not legally permit the practice of that belief.[45] Holding the belief is certainly legally permitted. I do not know whether Dworkin agrees with the Supreme Court decisions to which footnote 45 refers, but they illustrated the distinction between beliefs and practices as recognized in law. It would be one thing to believe in child sacrifice; it would be quite another to practice it. I do not expect that Dworkin, however tolerant of another's religious beliefs, would wish to have such a practice legally permitted. People, as Dworkin knows, are not free to follow their consciences when it comes to killing others or helping others kill themselves. We have abolished such practices as dueling, for example, a practice in which people defended their honor or dignity. Nor can people avenge a wrong they have suffered by killing the perpetrator, even when their cause is just. Rather, as a society, we say we believe in the rule of law in such matters.

And so the question before us is whether we also accept the rule of law when it comes to PAS and euthanasia, or whether we think it is a matter for individual consciences, rather than the common morality as now embedded in law.

As we noted earlier, the American Bar Association, in its Model Penal Code of 1980, took the view that the sanctity or sacredness of human life is threatened by those who would willingly participate in any act that would take the life of another individual, even if the individual who commits suicide requests that participation. How is such a threat best understood? As indicated earlier as well, in current law a human life is sacred in the sense that its worth is incalculable, and the interest of the State in protecting it unqualified. Furthermore, the love of life is a natural phenomenon. Human beings who procreate, nurture, and protect one another are expressing such a love for life. But life is also protected by the strong inhibitions against killing and being killed. It would be extremely difficult to enforce the laws against homicide if human beings had no inhibitions against killing and/or were inclined to hate life, their own and that of others.

Having just laws and order in a community is extremely important. In a situation in which law and order have broken down, individuals who have some hatreds or are seeking revenge may well overcome their usual inhibitions against killing. Once they do, their sense of the worth of a human life,

---

45. Polygamy, and the relevant Supreme Court decisions regarding this practice, are discussed in Mary Ann Glendon, *The Transformation of Family Law: State, Law, and Family in the United States and Western Europe* (Chicago: University of Chicago Press, 1989), pp. 52-55.

their own and that of others, may decline markedly, or even disappear. Consider the following account, gleaned in an interview of a Bosnian Serb sniper who killed Muslims in Sarajevo during the conflict there in the early years of the past decade. His name is Pipo. He claims to have killed 325 people. He tells the interviewer:

> All I know how to do is kill. I am not sure I am normal anymore. I can talk to people, but if someone pushes me, I will kill them. . . . In the beginning, I was able to put my fear aside, and it was good. Then with the killings, I was able to put my emotions aside, and it was good. But now they are gone.[46]

Pipo used to run a restaurant with a Muslim as his partner. That was before the war. Pipo joined the Bosnian Serb army but his hatred for Muslims did not begin until after his mother was jailed and beaten by them. In his words, "When she got out she wouldn't talk about it. That's when I picked up a gun and started shooting Muslims. I hate them all."[47] An officer in the sniper unit he joined taught him a useful mental technique to help him carry out his task: He told Pipo not to let the faces of those he shoots "follow him." Pipo learned to do his work well but he lost all of his normal feelings, even feelings of affection for his mother, the feelings that first drove him to avenge her victimization. Again, in Pipo's own words:

> I have no feelings for what I do. . . . I went to see my mother in Belgrade, and she hugged me and I felt nothing. . . . It is our choice to go to hell. . . . I have no life anymore. I go from day to day, but nothing means anything. I don't want a wife and children. I don't want to think.[48]

As reported, the interview with Pipo concludes after Pipo sends a visitor a note and some cigarettes to take to a friend who is a Muslim sniper and his opponent in the war. When he is asked whether he would kill that Muslim if he got him in the sights of his gun, he simply replied, "Why not?"[49]

This is a rather graphic account of an individual who has lost the love of life, and the proclivities and inhibitions that nourish and sustain it. Life has consequently no worth to him; neither his own, nor that of others. The sacredness of life has effectively no meaning for him. He calls the continuation of his life as a killer his own choice. Would Dworkin grant Pipo "freedom of conscience" for the choices he is making? I think not.

46. "A Sniper's Tale," *Time*, March 19, 1994, p. 24.
47. "A Sniper's Tale," *Time*, March 19, 1994, p. 24.
48. "A Sniper's Tale," *Time*, March 19, 1994, p. 24.
49. "A Sniper's Tale," *Time*, March 19, 1994, p. 24.

Dworkin could consider this story an extreme one, but it illustrates what can and does happen when the inhibitions against killing weaken sufficiently. In the initial government study of euthanasia as practiced in the Netherlands, physicians reported that, contrary to the legal rules governing the practice of it, they sometimes ended the lives of competent patients who had not requested euthanasia. The major reasons given were that the quality of life of these patients was very low and their families could not stand it any longer.[50] If such physicians still retained strong inhibitions against killing, they would surely want their competent patients to tell them how they believe their lives should end, and whether they believe the sacredness of life can still be upheld by them were they to request and receive euthanasia or assisted suicide.

Even the inhibition against killing animals, particularly pets, can be weakened. A veterinarian confided in me that she had a difficult struggle, emotionally, to give a lethal injection to a dog under her care even though doing it had the consent of the owners and it seemed to her a merciful thing to do. But, after administering euthanasia to a number of pet animals in the course of her practice, she had a shocking thought one day: She was killing these animals without any of the hesitations and emotional regrets she had felt when she did it for the first time.[51]

What I have been arguing is that the sacredness of life is a term that describes the worth of all individual human life as incalculable. Human beings naturally have the proclivities and inhibitions that sustain this idea of life's worth and the love for it. The laws against homicide are an expression of the community's interest, through its laws, to maintain the proclivities and inhibitions that render it at all possible to retain the sacredness of life as a standard of conduct and as a reality of communal life. After all, nurturing and protecting life are moral requisites of individual and communal life. Permitting in law the willingness to ask others to kill oneself, and the willingness to honor such a request, directly sanctions acts and practices that overcome the inhibitions against killing and the proclivity to nurture life, in oneself and others. To qualify what it means to call life sacred is to qualify or render contingent the incalculable worth of each individual life. If the law permits people to act on the premise that a life may not be worth living, by what moral principle and by what law does one prevent suicide and homicide? By what moral principle does one say that any deeply held wish to kill or be killed is a

50. See R. Fenigsen, "The Report of the Dutch Governmental Committee on Euthanasia," *Issues in Law and Medicine* 10, no. 2 (Fall 1994): 123-68.

51. Lisa Fullam, personal communication.

violation of the sacredness of human life that is the standard for protecting all individual human lives?

Dworkin would reply that it is possible to limit the freedom to kill and to assist in a suicide. Recognizing a need to limit assisted suicide, Dworkin, along with five other moral philosophers, suggested the following:

> A state might assert, for example, that people who are not terminally ill, but who have formed a desire to die, are, as a group, very likely later to be grateful if they are prevented from taking their own lives. It might then be legitimate, out of concern for such people, to deny them a doctor's assistance.[52]

Interestingly enough, this proposal, indirectly at least, acknowledges a general love of life, and the desirability of retaining some support for it in law. If Dworkin is assuming that individuals generally love their own lives, then he is claiming that terminal illness can be expected to undermine the love of life and render life unworthy of life, at least for some people. But only when caregivers and lawgivers act on the assumption that the terminally ill will be grateful for life once they are properly cared for, does the opportunity for that gratitude emerge for those terminally ill individuals who had been expressing a wish to die.

As discussed in Chapter One, Dr. Herbert Hendin, an American psychiatrist, has called attention to the powerful influence of physicians in the decisions of patients who are gravely or terminally ill.[53] In his analysis of the case of Diane, he noted the ways in which Dr. Timothy Quill aided his patient not only to carry out her death by suicide, but also influenced her to make that very decision.[54] Reacting to the considerable data on the practice of euthanasia in the Netherlands, Hendin has concluded that: "Euthanasia, fought for on the basis of the principle of autonomy and self-determination of patients, has actually increased the paternalistic power of the medical profession."[55] The Dutch physician, Dr. Herbert Cohen, is quoted by Dr. Hendin as saying, "Death is influenced by a doctor's decision in almost all nontraumatic cases. Death is an orchestrated happening."[56] That the doctor is "the conductor of the orchestra" has aroused concern among even the most avid supporters of

52. "Brief of Ronald Dworkin et al.," p. 196.

53. Herbert Hendin, "Seduced by Death: Doctors, Patients and the Dutch Cure," *Issues in Law and Medicine* 10, no. 2 (Fall 1994): 123-68.

54. Hendin, "Seduced by Death," pp. 125-28. For the case of Diane, see Timothy Quill, "Death and Dignity: A Case of Individualized Decision Making," *New England Journal of Medicine* 324, no. 10 (March 7, 1991): 691-94.

55. Hendin, "Seduced by Death," p. 163.

56. Hendin, "Seduced by Death," p. 160.

assisted suicide and euthanasia: They are becoming aware of too many physicians who are unaware of how the moods and wishes of patients can fluctuate, moods and wishes that can change during the course of treatment.[57]

The influence over how patients view their lives and whether they decide to end it does not stop with terminally ill patients. Patients who are not terminally ill can be persuaded to view their illness in such a way that they react to it as though it were a terminal illness. Dr. Richard Fenigsen, long a medical practitioner in the Netherlands, reported just such a case.[58] The patient, Mrs. P, was a seventy-two-year-old widow with a heart condition that responded well to treatment. She was living independently, though she needed help to keep her house clean, and her exercise was limited to walking a few blocks. She did sometimes come in with symptoms but they were successfully dealt with. Dr. Fenigsen described Mrs. P as "an extremely nice, mild-tempered lady who never showed any impatience and complied with the doctor's every order and advice."[59] When Mrs. P failed to appear at the outpatient clinic as expected, Dr. Fenigsen contacted her family physician, who told him that

> He had had a talk with Mrs. P . . . and explained the situation to her: This wasn't going to be any better, and living such a limited life, with all those pills, made no sense at all. Mrs. P accepted everything he said, he stopped her pills, and three days later she died.[60]

Fenigsen said that he was overcome by deep sorrow and that it returns every time he thinks of Mrs. P. She could have lived considerably longer.

Fenigsen assures the reader that this is not an isolated case of physicians convincing patients that they should die and then acting to end their lives. He cited the following data published by the Dutch Government Committee on Euthanasia:

> In 1990 about 86,000 people died while under medical care, and in 49,000 of these cases (57%) doctors at some point made decisions that could, or did, hasten deaths. In 14,550 cases the (medically not futile) life-prolonging treatment was withdrawn or withheld with intention to terminate life. Sixty-five percent of family physicians believe that doctors may propose (active) euthanasia to a patient who does not ask for it himself.[61]

57. Hendin, "Seduced by Death," p. 160.

58. Richard Fenigsen, "Physician-Assisted Death in the Netherlands: Impact on Long-Term Care," *Issues in Law and Medicine* 11, no. 3 (Winter 1995): 283-97.

59. Fenigsen, "Physician-Assisted Death in the Netherlands," p. 295.

60. Fenigsen, "Physician-Assisted Death in the Netherlands," p. 295.

61. Fenigsen, "Physician-Assisted Death in the Netherlands," p. 295.

From these cases and these data, we can observe that the beliefs of physicians regarding the sacredness of human life can influence and even shape the beliefs and actions of their patients. However intimate and personal end-of-life decisions may be, what these will be is much more dependent upon what others, particularly physicians, believe than Dworkin acknowledges. Dworkin unrealistically depicts individuals as quite disconnected from others with respect to what meaning and worth they give to their lives. What whole communities, loved ones, and physicians believe about the sacredness of individual human life has much more significance for each of us as individuals than Dworkin leads us to believe.

From these cases and these data we can observe that what the law has to say about the sacredness of life also influences and shapes the beliefs of patients and physicians. A complete ban on assisted suicide and euthanasia embodies in law the core of what it means to call life sacred; individual human life retains in principle its incalculable worth regardless of circumstances. It gives every individual and health professional a moral and legal reason to try to prevent suicide, as well as to alleviate any mental and/or physical distress that may tempt or drive someone to do it. However, if physicians and patients are legally permitted actively to kill, kill themselves, or assist others to kill themselves, some individuals, whether freely or under someone else's influence, will not have the opportunity to have their love of life sustained and supported in a way that inspires gratitude. And it was the potential for gratitude that Dworkin and his associates claimed should allow the states to deny physician assistance in a suicide. I agree that this is a reason for denying PAS, but I disagree that it applies only to individuals who are not terminally ill. It is a reason to deny PAS to everyone. As I have argued, people ought to be grateful for life, and ought to act in ways that help support the proclivities and inhibitions that sustain individual and communal life. And Dworkin does not give us any reason to believe that people will be grateful when they are prevented from committing suicide. He has implied but not affirmed that people do have a natural love of life, a love which, as I have indicated, expresses itself in the procreation, nurture, and protection of human life. This love is strong enough to yield an ever-growing number of people on this earth, despite all of the deaths that result from wars and natural disasters.

With regard to the consequences of permitting physicians to assist in suicide, Dworkin focuses exclusively on freedom of conscience for patients. As noted, this is a much more limited freedom than Dworkin hypothesizes. And, of course, ending one's life is the ultimate in destroying any freedom an individual may still retain while terminally or seriously ill. But Dworkin ignores what happens to physicians. They are free to follow their consciences on what they think is a life worth living, and free to influence people to act on their (the physicians') beliefs. Furthermore, the physicians themselves are partly, perhaps very strongly, swayed by what the law teaches them. This would appear to be the case in the Netherlands. Based on the data and his own experiences, Fenigsen is convinced that the growing preference for assisted suicide and euthanasia, even without requests for them, has mostly come after the courts there permitted physicians to honor requests for ending lives using lethal means.[62]

Dworkin has not provided a moral justification for preventing suicide, other than his appeal to gratitude: He has not, as I argued above, given us a reason to expect gratitude for having our lives saved. He does not explicitly affirm the natural love for life that would lead us to expect such gratitude.

Dworkin and his associates reject any suggestion of a slippery slope. But the German Constitutional Court responded self-consciously to the very idea that there is such a thing as a "life unworthy of life." They knew what actions accord with the belief that life is something less than an ultimate, incalculable value. Mindful also that the law is a teacher, the Court had this to say about how human life should be valued. Noting that Germany's Basic Law guarantees the protection of human dignity, the Court asserted that,

> Where human life exists, human dignity is present to it; it is not decisive that the bearer of this dignity himself be conscious of it and know personally how to preserve it.
> ... Human life represents within the order of the Basic Law, an ultimate value, the particulars of which need not be established; it is the living foundation of human dignity and the prerequisite for all other fundamental rights.[63]

These passages clearly express and support the idea that the worth of a life is incalculable: It comports with what I think it means to refer to life as sacred. And protecting human life, on this view, is at once a protection of human dignity at its core, and of all other rights, including individual freedom. Permitting PAS and euthanasia is compromising the freedom of many patients in the Netherlands and understandably so. In one sense, the freedom of all patients is compromised by permitting physicians to offer PAS. Offering PAS is something American laws on informed consent would undoubtedly require, if PAS were to be legally permitted.

---

62. Fenigsen, "Physician-Assisted Death in the Netherlands," p. 295.
63. "West German Abortion Decision," p. 419.

Concluding Reflections

I have argued that PAS and euthanasia, when practiced, violate the moral responsibility to treat human beings as having incalculable worth. Human life is sacred. I have also argued that all individuals have the inalienable right to have their lives so regarded and treated accordingly. This responsibility and this right are moral requisites of individual and communal life. These moral requisites are rendered possible by our natural proclivities to bring life into being and to nurture and protect it morally and legally. These moral requisites are rendered possible as well by our natural love of life and inhibitions against killing. Laws should help maintain, shape, and enforce these natural proclivities and inhibitions. To do this requires laws against homicide. To do this requires, as well, specific laws against assisted suicide and euthanasia.

That human life is sacred, that the love of life is natural, and that human beings have an inalienable right to life are affirmations embedded in law. All of these notions of human life were invoked in the United States Supreme Court's decisions to uphold the constitutionality of laws that totally prohibit assisted suicide.[64] These notions reflect a synthesis of traditions: the biblical and theological traditions in support of natural responsibilities to nurture and protect life and its sacredness; the Hobbesian and Lockean traditions of a natural, inalienable right to life. Hobbes and Locke also assert a natural desire of individuals to seek the preservation of their own lives. This constitutes a particular doctrine of human nature, however, and I have not based any of my own arguments on a particular concept of human nature or a particular theological anthropology, though the reader can certainly infer one from the account given of our natural proclivities and inhibitions. Elsewhere, I have discussed extensively why the courts and legislative bodies do not need to base laws against assisted suicide on a particular view of human nature.[65] In this same work, I indicate that, when proponents of PAS argue the moral neutrality of legally allowing individuals to decide for themselves whether to request PAS, they suppress the two traditions now embedded in law; that is hardly a neutral position.[66]

The idea of the sanctity or sacredness of life is not confined to the constitutional reasoning found, as we noted, in American and German courts. Consider this reasoning of the Supreme Court of Canada in its decision

---

64. *Washington v. Glucksberg* and *Vacco v. Quill.*

65. Arthur J. Dyck, *When Killing Is Wrong: Physician-Assisted Suicide and the Courts* (Cleveland: Pilgrim Press, 2001).

66. Dyck, *When Killing Is Wrong.*

(1993) to uphold the constitutionality of laws that completely prohibit assisted suicide. Writing for the majority, Judge Sopinka argued that protecting the "security of the person . . . cannot encompass a right to take action that will end one's life as security of the person is intrinsically concerned with the well-being of the living person."[67] Judge Sopinka spoke of this argument as one that "focuses on the generally held and deeply rooted belief in our society that human life is sacred or inviolable."[68] Taking up the issue of the purpose of laws that ban assisted suicide entirely, Judge Sopinka described the state interest in protecting life as a policy "that human life should not be depreciated by allowing life to be taken," and as a policy expressed in the *Criminal Code* prohibiting "murder and other violent acts against others, notwithstanding the consent of the victim."[69] But Judge Sopinka did not regard this as solely "a policy of the state" but as "part of our fundamental conception of the sanctity of human life."[70] He reviewed the policies of a number of nations and concluded that entirely banning assisted suicide is the norm for western democracies.[71]

Judge Sopinka expressly indicated that when he invoked the term "sacred," he was using the term in a nonreligious sense, namely, "to mean that human life is seen to have a deep intrinsic value of its own."[72] Similarly, I wish to make it clear, if it is not already abundantly clear, that I have used the term "sacred" in a nonreligious sense as well: to say that human life is sacred means that life is of incalculable worth. This concept of life's sacredness is compatible with Christian biblical and theological ways of thinking about life's worth.

But no one should mistake what I mean by considering the account I have given of life's sacredness as compatible with affirmations within the Christian tradition. Nothing in this book constitutes an appeal to authority as such. What I have tried to do throughout is to present reasoned arguments, appropriate to a public debate, for concepts and viewpoints currently embedded in law. I have sought to legitimate these from a moral perspective defended on the basis of reasoned arguments, relying upon logic and facts. No one need accept the traditions that have helped to shape the viewpoints and moral concepts currently embedded in law. But if my arguments are persuasive, anyone could, on rational and empirical grounds, accept the kind of moral structure that serves to undergird laws that prohibit assisted suicide

67. *Rodriguez v. British Columbia*, 107 D.L.R. 4th (1993), 389.
68. *Rodriguez v. British Columbia*, 107 D.L.R. 4th (1993), 389.
69. *Rodriguez v. British Columbia*, 107 D.L.R. 4th (1993), 396.
70. *Rodriguez v. British Columbia*, 107 D.L.R. 4th (1993), 396.
71. *Rodriguez v. British Columbia*, 107 D.L.R. 4th (1993), 404.
72. *Rodriguez v. British Columbia*, 107 D.L.R. 4th (1993), 389.

and euthanasia. In turn, I welcome reasoned criticism from my readers and anyone else, so that together we may come as close to the truth as possible on a subject that can surely divide people of good will. There is no exit from the necessity to forge policy that involves the protection of individual lives and to decide what laws are requisite for achieving that purpose.

Having made the claim that my portrayal of life's sacredness is compatible with affirmations found within the Christian tradition, I should consider whether that claim can be defended. There are some who may wish to contest that claim. Furthermore, why do I make this claim and why do I think it is important to defend it? Indeed, why be concerned at all with questions about the extent to which the central concepts and mode of defending them in this book are compatible with Christian beliefs and the bases for holding them? These are questions I now wish to address in the following and concluding chapter.

CHAPTER FOUR

Christian Morality and Natural Morality in Law and Public Policy

I n the previous chapter, I offered an account of what I called "the moral structure of life's worth and protection." As presented there, the structure of life's worth and protection expresses itself in at least three ways: as an individual, natural, and inalienable right to life; as a natural love of life; and as a belief in life's sacredness, that is, in its incalculable worth. These are naturally occurring phenomena. As human beings we have natural proclivities to bring life into being and to nurture and protect it; we also have inhibitions against killing ourselves and others. These proclivities and inhibitions find their sustenance in our natural love of life. These proclivities and inhibitions are requisites of individual and communal life and as such, essential ingredients in the natural morality we share as human beings. They provide the moral basis for homicide law. The concepts of an inalienable right to life, the natural love of life, and life's sacredness are present in constitutional law and, as noted previously, are to be found in the decisions of the United States Supreme Court to uphold the constitutionality of the laws of New York and Washington, totally prohibiting assisted suicide.[1] The concept of life's sacredness or sanctity is present in the reasoning of courts in other countries, as is the defense of laws against assisted suicide.[2]

---

1. *Washington v. Glucksberg,* 117 S. Ct. 2258 (1997); *Vacco v. Quill,* 117 S.Ct. 2293 (1997).

2. Two examples of affirming life's sacredness can be found in the decision of the Federal Constitutional Court of West Germany, published in full as "West German Abortion Decision: A Contrast to Roe v. Wade?" Robert E. Jones and John D. Gorby, trans., *John Marshall Journal of Practice and Procedure* 9 (Spring 1976): 605-84, and in the decision of the Canadian Supreme Court, *Rodriguez v. British Columbia,* 1107 D.L.R. 4th 342 (1993). The Ca-

The moral structure of life's worth and protection is a vital segment of the natural morality shared by human beings and, as such, provides a principled basis for homicide law. Indeed, I have argued that this moral structure would be undermined, and rejected in principle, by policies that would legally permit PAS and euthanasia. I have also indicated that I regard this moral structure as compatible with affirmations found within the Christian tradition. In what respects this compatibility exists and why this compatibility is important to discuss and understand is the concern of this chapter.

To begin with, then, I will argue that within the Christian tradition there are substantive affirmations of the moral structure of life's worth and protection as it is being described and supported in this book, including its three major manifestations in a natural, inalienable right to life, a natural love of life, and the belief in life's sacredness. Secondly, I wish to indicate the importance of this for those who profess to be Christians and for those who do not. Nothing less than the sustenance of our common humanity and the democratic polity based upon it are at stake.

Christian Affirmations of the Moral Structure of Life's Worth

The Natural, Inalienable Right to Life

Every human being has an inalienable right to life: the American Declaration of Independence describes that as a self-evident truth. The French Declaration of Rights similarly affirms an individual right to life, describing it as natural and imprescriptable. The United Nations as well claims universality for human rights, viewing them as "characteristics of the human family" and as "equal and inalienable."[3] The right to life is among these.[4]

The natural and inalienable right to life is not only found in the American Declaration of Independence, but also in American constitutional law. Two traditions fed into the acceptance of and articulation of this right in America: The Christian and the Hobbesian/Lockean.[5] These two traditions achieved a

---

nadian court noted that Western democracies totally prohibit assisted suicide, and the U.S. Supreme Court quoted this finding in *Glucksberg,* footnote 8, p. 2263.

3. United Nations, *Universal Declaration of Human Rights,* (1949), "Preamble."
4. United Nations, *Universal Declaration of Human Rights,* (1949), "Article 3."
5. Within American political and legal history, ways of thinking associated with Christianity and with Hobbes and Locke qualify as traditions as I am using the term. A tradition is "an inherited, established, or customary pattern of thought." (See *Webster's Tenth New Collegiate Dictionary.*) These patterns of thought are "inherited" in the sense of being

synthesis that Max Stackhouse has described as the "Liberal-Puritan Synthesis."[6] This synthesis provided, and still provides, a rationale for Western democratic institutions, laws, and practices. Those, in the tradition of Hobbes and Locke, designated as "liberal" by Stackhouse, viewed natural, inalienable rights as rationally self-evident; Puritans viewed these same rights as divinely and rationally revealed truths. One can readily observe these two traditions within the American Declaration of Independence. The Puritan element is in the description of humans as "born equal," and the rights being articulated as "endowed by the Creator"; the Hobbesian/Lockean element is in the resort to the language of rights, to articulate that with which we humans have been endowed by God. For both traditions, these are natural possessions that cannot be taken away, hence, inalienable.

What Stackhouse called the "Liberal-Puritan Synthesis," I prefer to call the "Natural Rights Synthesis." This synthesis constitutes an acceptance by biblically informed Christians of the Hobbesian and Lockean description of the moral imperatives to protect life and liberty as natural, inalienable rights. This synthesis is so deeply ingrained that it can be invoked unself-consciously in scholarly reflections on the nature of Christian thought and influence. Consider, for example, the claim by Darrel W. Amundsen that "the Christian concept of the imago Dei provided both the basis and the structure of the idea of inalienable rights and intrinsic human values that has prevailed in Western society until the present."[7] Notice that Amundsen does not at all feel compelled to explain that the concept of "inalienable rights" has another, more recent source. It refers to Hobbes, who did not explicitly base the inalienable right to life on the "imago Dei" (hereafter, image of God) but rather on the egoistic, natural desire of human beings to preserve their own lives. It is Hobbes as well who began a mode of thinking that treats "rights" as a major, if not the major moral imperative of our shared, natural morality. Given what we know about Hobbes, it is not possible to establish how much, if at all, Hobbes was shaped

---

present for more than a generation; "established" in the sense of providing a rationale, sometimes implicitly and sometimes explicitly, for individual, institutional, and legal decisions; and "customary" in the sense of finding expression in conventional societal practices and individual actions.

6. Max Stackhouse, *Creeds, Society, and Human Rights: A Study in Three Cultures* (Grand Rapids: Eerdmans, 1984).

7. Darrel W. Amundsen, *Medicine, Society, and Faith in the Ancient and Medieval Worlds* (Baltimore: Johns Hopkins University Press, 1996). This claim comes in a section of the book entitled "The Christian Principle of the Sanctity of Life," to which I will refer further when discussing the sacredness of human life as a Christian belief. Note also that the imago Dei is an idea found in the biblical book of Genesis, a source of revelation for Jews to begin with, and only later for Christians.

or influenced by Christian ideas, such as the image of God. However, what we do know is that Hobbes did not offer an avowedly Christian argument for inalienable rights. We know also that it is by way of Hobbes and Locke that the concept of natural rights began its significant role in law and public policy.

Still, the citation from Amundsen identifies a biblical basis for embracing natural and inalienable rights as a way to characterize life's worth, and serves as a moral and legal rationale for life's protection. And, that is what the Puritans did. Furthermore, Amundsen has put his finger on an aspect of the right to life in law that appears to be Christian in its origin, or that is certainly a Christian way of thinking. The law's interest in preserving life is unqualified and is in no way contingent on an individual's characteristics or circumstances. This point we noted in Chapter Three. Amundsen makes this same point about the Christian affirmation of life's worth, its sacredness, by calling attention to the fact that Christians, unlike the Greek and Roman traditions, did not condone the practice of infanticide. As he observes, "the imago Dei, with its attendant value, rights, and responsibilities, attached in early Christian thought to the newborn, whether healthy or sickly, maimed, deformed or monstrous, indeed to the whole continuum of the defective, in vivid contrast to the attitudes and practices of pagan antiquity."[8] Clearly, the unconditional worth of human life is a Christian tenet. I once asked a class at Harvard Divinity School whether there is any moral outlook or practice influenced by some unique aspect of the Christian ethic. The class was hesitant to reply, but after a pause, it was a Buddhist monk and medical doctor who ventured an answer. In Thailand, the country in which he worked and in which he was born, this monk said that Christians had changed the attitudes of his people to regard persons with disabilities or handicaps of whatever sort favorably and to afford them the same respect and rights as all other members of society. Before Christians came to Thailand, he said, attitudes were very different. I turn now to examine the connection made in Christian thinking between the natural, inalienable right to life and life's sacredness, understood as life's incalculable worth.

Life's Sacredness

As the reader will recall, American constitutional law has spoken of the right to life, within common law, as both sacred and inalienable.[9] Since appeals to

8. Amundsen, *Medicine, Society, and Faith in the Ancient and Medieval Worlds.*

9. *Washington v. Glucksberg,* 2265. Note that courts use the terms "sacred" and "having sanctity" as synonymous.

the sacredness of life are widespread in Western law, it is not surprising to find Pope John Paul II asserting that the majority of human beings believe that life is sacred. Similarly, since the United Nations has enunciated a natural, universal right to life, it is also not surprising that Pope John Paul II would regard an attack on the life of innocent individuals, whether upon one's own life or that of another, as violating a fundamental right, a right that cannot be lost or alienated. This violation is one of the major reasons the Pope considers both homicide and intentional death, that is, suicide, as wrong.[10] Whatever the origins of incorporating into law the idea that life is both an inalienable, natural right and sacred, Christians, in whatever number, clearly have affirmed, and do now affirm, life's worth in this way. This is true, then, of the Roman Catholic appropriation of Christian beliefs, as well as that of Protestants. As we have already noted the Puritans were a case in point. A major source of Puritan thought, and that of Protestants more generally, is John Calvin. I wish to dwell briefly on his thinking to illustrate further the significance of the image of God within the Christian tradition, as a basis for life's worth.

In his major work, *Institutes of the Christian Religion,* Calvin devotes a full chapter to an explanation of the "moral law," the contents of which he equates with the Ten Commandments.[11] Although Calvin uses the terms "man" and "men" throughout his discussion of the image of God, he clearly believed that men and women, as the first chapter of Genesis indicated, are both created in God's image.[12] Hence, what he has to say about the commandment against killing applies equally to men and women.[13] Calvin views the purpose of this commandment as binding humanity together, creating unity. Therefore, every individual ought to be concerned "with the safety of all."[14] This involves much more than the avoidance of killing:

10. Pope John Paul II, *Euthanasia: Declaration of the Sacred Congregation for the Doctrine of the Faith* (May 5, 1980). The reader can find this document in *The Pope Speaks* (Winter, 1980): 289-96. It is reprinted in Stephen E. Lammers and Allen Verhey, eds., *On Moral Medicine: Theological Perspectives in Medial Ethics* (Grand Rapids: Eerdmans, 1998), pp. 650-54.

11. John Calvin, *Institutes of Christian Religion,* ed. John T. McNeil, trans. Ford Lewis Battles (Philadelphia: Westminster Press, 1960), II, VIII, 367-423.

12. For an interesting account of Calvin's view of women, and how far his affirmation of their natural equality changed their status in the church and in society, see Jane Dempsey Douglass, *Women, Freedom and Calvin* (Philadelphia: Westminster Press, 1985).

13. In the *Institutes,* the sixth commandment is translated "You shall not kill" (Exod. 20:13). Some translations offer both "murder" and "kill" as possible translations of the biblical text. (See NRSV.)

14. Calvin, *Institutes,* II, VIII, 39, 404.

77

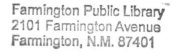

To sum up, then, all violence, injury, and any harmful thing to all that may injure our neighbor's body are forbidden to us. We are accordingly commanded, if we find anything of use to us in saving our neighbors' lives, faithfully to employ it; if there is anything that makes for their peace to see to it; if anything harmful, to ward it off; if they are in any danger, to lend a helping hand.[15]

In Calvin's summary, one can observe the moral responsibilities that serve as the impetus and rationale for a number of contemporary communal institutions, regulations, and laws. Beyond the existence of armed forces and a civilian police force, there are provisions for firefighting, regulations and laws regarding the safety in food and in the workplace, laws to protect against toxicity in the environment, the licensing and oversight of the healing professions and institutions, a variety of public health measures and organizations, and in many nations, a legal duty to rescue. Such a list is not exhaustive. Children are protected in special ways by laws encouraging nurture and protecting against neglect and abuse. In all of the efforts, one can see that they all ultimately seek to prevent death insofar as that is possible. Even in simpler communities, past and present, there are analogies to these same organized efforts.

Calvin provides the following reason for these moral imperatives encompassed in the moral imperative not to kill:

Scripture notes that this commandment rests upon a twofold basis: man is both the image of God, and our flesh. Now if we do not wish to violate the image of God, we ought to hold our neighbor sacred. And if we do not wish to renounce all humanity, we ought to cherish his as our own flesh. . . . The Lord has willed that we consider these two things which are naturally in man, and might lead us to seek his preservation: to reverence his image imprinted in man, and to embrace our own flesh in him.[16]

Note how Calvin links the sacredness of human beings to the image of God with which each individual is naturally endowed. A failure to seek the preservation of human life is at once a violation of the image of God and that individual's sacredness; it is a failure to reverence God's imprinted image in one's neighbor.

This reverence for the image of God should not depend upon how we value a fellow human being, nor upon any of their merit or lack thereof. The worth of individual life that ought to ground our own behavior is beyond all

---

15. Calvin, *Institutes*, II, VIII, 39, 404.
16. Calvin, *Institutes*, II, VIII, 40, 404-5.

evaluation; it is invaluable. Interestingly enough, the explicit affirmation of the incalculable worth of human life occurs in the context of Calvin's explanation of what it means to love our neighbor which is, after all, the sum and essence of what is required of us by the moral law. Doing good for one's neighbor is exceptionless. If merit were to be the basis for doing good, few would qualify in Calvin's view. Rather, we are to look to the image of God in everyone, to that "which we owe all honor and love."[17] When we do that, we will have no reason to refuse help to anyone who needs it. As Calvin puts it,

> Say, "He is contemptible and worthless"; but the Lord shows him to be one to whom he has deigned to give the beauty of his image.... Say that he does not deserve even your best effort for his sake; but the image of God which recommends him to you, is worthy of giving yourself and all your possessions.[18]

Yet, what about Calvin's other basis for preserving human life? I refer to "embracing our own flesh" in the person of our neighbor. It is in this very discussion of love of neighbor that Calvin explicates what that implies. Calvin perceives that individuals may recognize the invaluable worth of human beings, but yet not feel responsible to render aid to everyone they meet that is in need. Calvin confronts, as a possible exception to rendering such aid, that the individual is a stranger to you. His reply to that is to point out that every stranger has been given by the Lord "a mark that ought to be familiar to you by virtue of the fact that he forbids you to despise your own flesh," and to refer the reader to Isaiah 58:7.[19] In this biblical text, the prophet Isaiah is indicating some of the actions, among others, that count as practicing righteousness. "Is it not," he declares, "to share your bread with the hungry and bring the homeless poor into your house; when you see the naked to cover them, and not to hide yourself from your own kin?" (NRSV). In short, as human beings, we share a body; the bodily needs of others are as familiar as our own. The injunction not to kill includes a moral responsibility to endeavor to preserve the lives of ourselves and of others by meeting all bodily needs — in a word, "to embrace our own flesh," in us and in others. One cannot, and should not, separate the image of God from its fleshly embodiment. This is what I interpret Calvin as saying to us. Hence, Calvin is saying as well that there is a basis for reverencing human life, as we know it here on earth, as sacred and of incalculable worth.

17. Calvin, *Institutes,* III, VII, 6, 696.
18. Calvin, *Institutes,* III, VII, 6, 696.
19. Calvin, *Institutes,* III, VII, 6, 696.

Christian descriptions of human life as having an incalculable worth are by no means confined to the past. The twentieth-century Protestant theologian Helmut Thielicke, whose work has resonance within the contemporary literature of bioethics, is but one example.[20] Thielicke has suggested two ways in which to view individual human beings: From the standpoint of their utility, or from the standpoint of their "infinite worth."[21] What he characterizes as the "incommensurable, incalculable worth of human life" is due to the image of God in us.[22] God's image results from God's love as our Creator and Redeemer.[23]

There is at least one contemporary Christian ethicist who appears to be questioning the claim that the concept of life's sacredness, certainly as I have depicted it in Chapter Three and now in Calvin, is at all a Christian belief, or at all compatible with the Christian tradition as he, Stanley Hauerwas, understands it. Hauerwas has confidently declared that "Christians certainly do not believe that life is inherently sacred and therefore it must be sustained until the bitter end."[24] What this assertion means needs to be put into context. In the paragraph preceding this denial that life is inherently sacred, Hauerwas is making a case for a responsibility shared by all those who are sick and being cared for. "That responsibility," he tells us, "is simply to keep on living."[25] He characterizes this obligation as follows:

> It is an obligation that we at once owe to our Creator and one another. For our creaturely status is but a reminder that our existence is not secured by our own power, but rather requires the constant care of, and trust in, others. Our willingness to live in the face of suffering, pain, and sheer boredom of life is morally a service to one another as it is a sign that life can be endured and moreover our living can be done with joy and exuberance.[26]

20. See Karen Lebacqz, "Alien Dignity: The Legacy of Helmut Thielicke for Bioethics," first published in 1996, reprinted in Lammers and Verhey, eds., *On Moral Medicine*, pp. 184-92.

21. Helmut Thielicke, "The Doctor as Judge of Who Shall Live and Who Shall Die," in Kenneth Vaux, ed., *Who Shall Live? Medicine, Technology, Ethics* (Philadelphia: Fortress Press, 1970).

22. Thielicke, "The Doctor as Judge," p. 170.

23. Thielicke, "The Doctor as Judge," p. 170. Thielicke refers to our worth as "alien dignity," that is, as a worth derived from God and our relationship to God.

24. Stanley Hauerwas, *Suffering Presence: Theological Reflections on Medicine, the Mentality of the Handicapped, and the Church* (Notre Dame: University of Notre Dame Press, 1986), p. 106.

25. Hauerwas, *Suffering Presence*, p. 106.

26. Hauerwas, *Suffering Presence*, p. 106.

Having posited a continuous responsibility to live as a moral service to others, he wishes the reader to know that "there is nothing about this position which entails that we must do everything we can to keep ourselves alive under all conditions."[27] So far this account is not one that I see as differing in any significant way from my own portrayal of a continuous responsibility to live in a way that signifies gratitude for the procreation, nurture, and protection of our lives owed to others, and thereby provide encouragement to others to retain their love of life and inhibition against killing. That we owe gratitude to our Creator is something I also affirm. I have chosen, however, to base my arguments against requesting assisted suicide or euthanasia on purely nonreligious grounds and so I have come to a view similar to that of Hauerwas without explicitly invoking our debt to God by reason of being created by God. And, like Hauerwas, I have distinguished comfort-only treatment that may compromise the length of our lives, from taking one's own life, or having it taken, by lethal means. But Hauerwas seems to find the position we essentially share incompatible with a belief in the "inherent sacredness of life," a belief moreover that he does not think any Christians hold. How am I to respond to that since I claim that my concept of life's sacredness is compatible with what I take to be a Christian way of thinking about life?

It is not entirely clear to me what Hauerwas is denying when he denies that life is, as he puts it, "inherently sacred." One partial clue is found in the assertion that immediately follows this denial of life's sacredness: "The existence of martyrs is a clear sign that Christians think the value of life can be overridden."[28] To begin with then, the question being posed for me is whether the belief in the sacredness of life, meaning that life is of incalculable worth, is a belief that would regard martyrdom as generally, or in all cases, a morally unjustifiable violation of life's incalculable worth. I will limit any discussion to two kinds of martyrdom, without claiming that these are exhaustive of all possible morally justifiable instances of martyrdom.

Among the first Christian martyrs were those who died at the hands of Roman officials because they would not renounce their Christian faith. Accepting as I do that the responsibility to live is owed to God, as well as other human beings, the willingness to die rather than repudiate one's Christian beliefs is a decision not simply to die but to meet one's responsibility to maintain one's relationship to God, and thereby maintain one's hold on eternal life. To die as a result of affirming a life that, if properly lived, is eternal, is not a denial of the incalculable worth of one's life. It is the one who kills the

27. Hauerwas, *Suffering Presence,* p. 106.
28. Hauerwas, *Suffering Presence,* p. 106.

Christian who is denying the incalculable worth of that individual's life. How that Christian is related to God and to the possibility of eternal life is for God to judge. For Christians, the choice to live affirming their reliance on God as long as they are physically able is a choice to live eternally even if, and even when to do so means being put to death. I would not characterize this, as Hauerwas does, as an example of "overriding the value of life" nor of violating the notion that life is sacred in the sense of having incalculable worth. Indeed, in the case under discussion, these martyrs valued life so much that when they are forced to choose, they choose life that lasts forever over life that does not. These martyrs are witnessing to their belief that Jesus is "the resurrection and the life," and their belief that all individuals "who believe in [Jesus], even though they die will live."[29] Provided that a Christian is witnessing to this faith and not seeking to escape from life's responsibilities on earth, they die affirming rather than denying life's incalculable worth.

In his book, *Death by Choice*, the Christian ethicist Daniel Maguire has suggested that the Christian belief "that death does not end life," helps justify PAS and euthanasia under certain circumstances:

> For a Christian and for anyone who believes in an afterlife, to "terminate life" is not to terminate life, but to move on to a new life. . . . This would seem to make it easier for a Christian to see death as a friend, especially when he or she has, through illness, lost all ability to respond and react to the invitation of his God to join him in the building up of this earth.[30]

But contrary to what Maguire is claiming, both Hauerwas and I agree that those who are ill and dying, whatever their condition, can and should render one last service to their companions on earth, namely to refrain from requesting or having others request, on their behalf, PAS or euthanasia. I will not repeat the extensive arguments for viewing this service as a definite moral and legal responsibility. Suffice it to say at this point that it is a responsibility that contributes to "building up" life on earth for others by strengthening the proclivities and inhibitions that create and sustain human life; it is also a responsibility both for those who believe in an afterlife, and for those who do not.

As we have noted, Christians may become martyrs for refusing to renounce their faith. There is another way in which individuals, whether Chris-

---

29. John 11:25-26 (NRSV).
30. Daniel C. Maguire, *Death by Choice* (Garden City, N.Y.: Doubleday, 1984), pp. 129-30. For a view opposing suicide and depicting death as both friend and foe, see Dennis P. Hollinger, "A Theology of Death," in Timothy J. Demy and Gary P. Stewart, eds., *Suicide: A Christian Response* (Grand Rapids: Kregel, 1998), pp. 257-67.

tian or not, may voluntarily act to relinquish, or risk relinquishing, their lives. They may lay down their lives for another — a parent, for example, may seek to rescue a son or daughter from a burning building at the risk of dying in the attempt. Even if the parent dies in such an instance, this action in no way signals to anyone that life is not of incalculable worth. On the contrary, the act signals just the opposite. Only if the smoke and heat of the fire is so intense that no one could possibly survive it long enough to rescue anyone would the endeavor to do so be regarded as suicidal. Indeed, in such circumstances bystanders have restrained would-be rescuers from needlessly losing their lives.

One could give many different actual and imagined instances in which a life is risked or lost for the sake of saving one or more other lives that cannot be saved in any other way. In such instances, the value of life is not being overridden. In short, martyrdom that is not sought for its own sake can involve actions that are consistent with the affirmation of life's sacredness.

From a Christian biblical point of view, human beings have been created in the image of God, blessed by God at creation, and regarded by God as "very good."[31] For this reason alone one can surely say that God has rendered human life "sacred," endowing it with a worth that human beings cannot even fathom let alone calculate. However, there are other reasons, from a Christian biblical perspective, for affirming the incalculable worth of human life. The twentieth-century Christian theologian, Karl Barth, has called attention to the fact of the incarnation as the best answer to the question as to why life is to be respected. In contrast to finding respect for life by resort to "general religious expressions," nature, or reason, Barth asserts that "the respect of life which becomes a command in the recognition of the union of God with humanity in Jesus Christ has an incomparable power and width."[32] Once the focus is on Christ, however, there are still further reasons to have an unqualified regard for life's worth. For one thing, Christ died so that all human beings have the possibility of not perishing, but having eternal life.[33] What is more, Christ not only took on human flesh and died, but was also raised from death as a human being. This resurrection became the basis for putting an end to death: "For since death came through a human being, the resurrection of the dead has also come through a human being; for as all die in Adam, so all will be made alive in Christ."[34]

The Christian ethicist, the late Paul Ramsey, reminded all those who were

31. Genesis 1:26-31 (NRSV).
32. Karl Barth, *Church Dogmatics*, III/4, trans. A. T. Mackay et al. (Edinburgh: T. & T. Clark, 1961), p. 339.
33. John 15:26-31 (NRSV).
34. 1 Corinthians 15:21-22 (NRSV).

advocating death with dignity why it is important to retain the biblical view that death is the ultimate enemy: The tendency of modern times is to deny the tragedy of death, in ways that have the effect of reducing the unique worth and "once-for-all-ness" of the "individual life-span" lost through death.[35] Responding favorably to Paul Ramsey, the Christian ethicist Oliver O'Donovan also asserts "the importance of the individual as an irreplaceable bearer of human value."[36] There is a Christian basis for viewing individuals as irreplaceable. As O'Donovan observes, "the resurrection grounds the eternal value of the individual."[37] From a Christian standpoint, death is a defeated enemy; it is the life of every individual that has imperishable worth. I can do no better than remind the reader of this stirring affirmation in words many have heard and many have sung, found in Scripture and in Handel's "Messiah,"

> Listen, I will tell you a mystery! We will not all die, but we will all be changed, in a moment, in the twinkling of an eye, at the last trumpet. For the trumpet will sound, and the dead will be raised imperishable. For this perishable body must put on imperishability, and this mortal body must put on immortality. When this perishable body puts on imperishability, and this mortal body puts on immortality, then the saying that is written will be fulfilled: "Death has been swallowed up in victory." "Where, O death, is your victory? Where, O death, is your sting?" The sting of death is sin. . . . But thanks be to God who gives us the victory through our Lord Jesus Christ.[38]

Surely the Christian belief in the resurrection puts the worth of individual human life beyond all calculation. At the same time, the belief in the resurrection puts the extent of God's love beyond all calculation. In choosing to follow the resurrected Christ, Christians choose life, not death, in this life, and in the life to come.

The Natural Love of Life

As noted above, and also in Chapter Three, the United States Supreme Court explicitly recognized a natural love of life in its unanimous decision to reject

35. Paul Ramsey, "The Indignity of 'Death with Dignity,'" Hastings Center Studies 2 (May 1974): 47-62.

36. Oliver O'Donovan, "Keeping Body and Soul Together," in Lammers and Verhey, eds., On Moral Medicine, p. 233.

37. O'Donovan, "Keeping Body and Soul Together," p. 235.

38. 1 Corinthians 15:51-57 (NRSV).

physician-assisted suicide as a constitutional right.[39] Laws against assisted suicide presume that there is a positive desire to live and where it is temporarily lost, individuals need to be protected by law, and, when seriously ill and in pain, should receive the care that will restore the desire to live. These points are also found in the U.S. Supreme Court decision regarding assisted suicide, including a reference to patients who had been suicidal, and who, once treated for depression and pain, are "grateful to be alive."[40] Without laws against assisted suicide, some individuals requesting suicide would not have the opportunity to have their love of life restored. The need for such opportunities clearly exists. Research indicates that 95 percent of those who committed suicide had a major psychiatric illness at the time.[41] For some psychiatrists, desiring to commit suicide should always be regarded as a condition that should receive psychiatric intervention.[42]

However, as noted also in Chapter Three, whatever the extent to which the loss of love of one's own life may be associated with mental illness, losing love for one's life does impair moral cognition. In his definition of what it means to be a friend to someone, Aristotle included the wish that the other person exist and live as mothers do in relation to their children.[43] For Aristotle, knowing how to be a friend to someone depends upon knowing how to relate to ourselves. Those who know that it is loving to wish life for another are those who love their own lives, that is, who wish to exist. To love another individual's life is part of what it means to be a friend to that individual. Aristotle's reference to maternal love provides his readers with some evidence that human beings have both the natural proclivity and natural knowledge to relate properly to themselves and hence, to others. In effect, human beings all have the capacity and knowledge to practice the Golden Rule, and hence, to be friends to one another.

What Aristotle did in finding a natural basis for the affirmation of our own lives and those of others has its parallel in the version of the Golden Rule recorded in the Gospel of Matthew: The overall setting for this is the Sermon on the Mount. Immediately preceding the reference to the Golden Rule is an invitation by Jesus to ask things of God, and a promise that such requests will be honored (Matthew 7:7-8). There, the Golden Rule is put into the context of divine and human parenthood as follows:

39. *Glucksberg*, 2264.

40. *Glucksberg*, 2272-73

41. *Glucksberg*, 2272.

42. See, for example, Peter Sainsbury, "Community Psychiatry," in Seymour Perlin, ed., *A Handbook for the Study of Suicide* (New York: Oxford University Press, 1975).

43. Aristotle, *Nichomachean Ethics*, Book IX, Chapter 4.

Which of you, if his son asks him for bread, will give him a stone? Or if he asks for a fish, will give him a snake? If you then, though you are evil, know how to give good gifts to your children, how much more will your father in heaven give good gifts to those who ask him? So in everything, do to others what you would have them do to you, for this sums up the Law and the Prophets. (Matthew 7:9-12, NIV)

In the Revised Standard Version of this passage, the Golden Rule is worded somewhat differently: "So whatever you wish that men should do to you, do to them" (Matthew 7:12). This wording makes the link to Aristotle even more transparent.

According to Matthew's account, Jesus, in this segment of the Sermon on the Mount, is asserting that parents naturally know what is good. In the examples given, parents wish to give their children what is necessary to sustain their lives, and they know what it takes to sustain their own lives. Jesus assumes that they wish life for themselves, for they would not wish life for their children if they did not wish life for themselves. Hence, the love of life, expressed in behavior that nurtures and protects human life, is a reliable natural guide for knowing what the moral law and its champions, the prophets, require of all of us. For one thing, the moral law, the Ten Commandments, forbid killing. The intentional failure to nurture and protect the lives of one's children would be as great a violation of the moral law as the actions that directly intend their deaths. In the context this provided for the Golden Rule in Matthew's Gospel, all human beings are expected to know the moral law, and to be mindful to act in accord with it. Parental behavior demonstrates the existence of such natural knowledge and natural inclinations. And these proclivities to bring life into being, and nurture and protect it, and the inhibitions against destroying life, are present in human beings despite the presence also within them of moral imperfections and sin. All human beings, then, are held responsible, without excuse, for living in accord with the Golden Rule. As we shall discuss later, doing this is an expression of the image of God within us, and our evil tendencies do not destroy this image and its potential for knowing and doing what is good.

At this point, it is important to emphasize again that the natural love of life is acknowledged in a very significant guide for Christian beliefs and practices — the biblical account of the Sermon on the Mount. Furthermore, to wish the self and the other to exist is at the very core of what it takes to know how to behave morally and to be inclined so to behave. Individuals who do not care whether they, or anyone else, live or die, no longer have a basis for being moral, or for desiring to be so. Without the wish that the self and the other exist, the Golden Rule is empty of any content that would protect human life; without the wish that the self and the others exist, there is no longer a reason to be moral. God, within Christianity, loves every individual human life. God created it. God rescued it. And God offers to sustain it eternally. God is the ultimate in parental love as this passage in Matthew also underlines.

As noted earlier, Karl Barth regards respect for life as something God has commanded of all human beings. To respect life is to stand in awe and wonder of it:

> And this means that human life must be affirmed and willed by man. We hasten to add that it must be affirmed and willed as his own with that of others and that of others with his own. . . . My own life can no more claim respect than that of others, but neither can that of others. Although they are not the same, but each distinct, the homogeneity and solidarity of all human life is indissoluble.[44]

In order to clarify further how the will to live is to be understood, Barth spells out further some of the specific human actions that express a determination and readiness to confirm life. For one thing, if our perception and confirmation of life is what it ought to be, "it must consist in our making of our life the use prescribed by its nature."[45] To do this responsibly requires that "we cannot and must not seriously tire of life."[46] Barth notes that a responsible use of our lives is always threatened by an egoism. The corrective for that is to recall that the real human life is to be "lived in orientation to God and coordination with others."[47] Living in "coordination" with others has particularly important practical import for Barth, because, as he says,

> The will to live which is the form of respect for life will always be distinguishable from an inhuman and irreverent will to live contrary to the command, by the fact that it considers the life of others together with its own, and its own together with that of others.[48]

Barth leaves us in no doubt that respect for life constitutes a will or wish that the self and the other live, and that such a commitment to life is a corrective for irresponsible use of our lives, and prescribed by its nature. Furthermore, respect for life, as willing one's own life and that of others, gives substance

44. Karl Barth, *Church Dogmatics*, III/IV, p. 341.
45. Karl Barth, *Church Dogmatics*, III/IV, p. 341.
46. Karl Barth, *Church Dogmatics*, III/IV, p. 341.
47. Karl Barth, *Church Dogmatics*, III/IV, p. 341.
48. Karl Barth, *Church Dogmatics*, III/IV, p. 341.

and guidance to the Golden Rule. Among other things, respect for life, for Barth, "consists in granting to the other the same as one grants to oneself," and, in this context, he is, as in the Sermon on the Mount, talking about what is necessary to sustain life.[49]

And so, in the Christian tradition there is clearly an affirmation of the natural love of life and of its role in making it possible for all human beings to know what is morally right. Undercutting our love of life undercuts the moral structure that protects all of our lives, by weakening or extinguishing both our desire to be moral and our ability to know what being moral entails. Wishing the self and the other to exist is a moral imperative for all human beings, for the reasons given in Chapter Three. From a Christian perspective, it is also a command of God, and as such, one that all human beings ought to heed, and one that all human beings are naturally capable of heeding. Furthermore, from a Christian perspective, this natural love of life came to be and persists because God has so created us and continues so to sustain us.

Sustaining Our Common Morality: A Shared Responsibility

So far, this chapter has illustrated and documented that the moral structure of life's worth undergirding homicide law is not only articulated within constitutional law, but also within explicitly Christian literature, both past and present. All of the major components of this moral structure can be discerned in Christian discussions of life's worth, namely that the worth of human life is incalculable, that the right to life is inalienable, and that there is a natural love of life, a love of one's own life and that of others. This should not be surprising to those who are aware that the Christian tradition provides a rationale for aspects of the moral life we naturally share as human beings. Cynthia B. Cohen, a contemporary philosopher and lawyer, writing about the Christian tradition, makes this very point as she urges that "as we develop a social consensus about assisted suicide and euthanasia, religious voices should be heard, for they share with secular voices an embedded common morality."[50]

Notice, however, that Cohen has introduced our common morality in the form of an argument for paying attention to what religious individuals and groups have to say about public policy regarding assisted suicide and eu-

---

49. Karl Barth, *Church Dogmatics,* III/IV, p. 347.
50. Cynthia B. Cohen, "Christian Perspectives on Assisted Suicide and Euthanasia: The Anglican Tradition," in Margaret P. Battin, Rosamond Rhodes, and Anita Silvers, eds., *Physician Assisted Suicide: Expanding the Debate* (New York: Routledge, 1998), p. 334.

thanasia. She does not take for granted that religious voices (she focuses upon Christian voices in this article) will be attended to sufficiently to help shape the direction and outcome of this debate. Her article is, among other things, an effort to gain a place in a new social consensus for ideas originating within the Christian tradition.

However, in her concern to "develop a social consensus" that would include religious and secular voices, she takes no notice that such a consensus now exists in law. Chief Justice Rehnquist, writing for the United States Supreme Court, called attention to over seven hundred years of "Anglo-American" law prohibiting assisted suicide, a prohibition extending into the present: "In almost every state — indeed, in almost every Western democracy — it is a crime to assist a suicide. The States' assisted suicide bans are not innovations. Rather, they are longstanding expressions of a State's commitment to the protection and preservation of all human life."[51] Citing a previous U.S. Supreme Court decision, Chief Justice Rehnquist indicated that the laws against assisted suicide constitute a "national consensus" because "'[T]he primary and most reliable indication of [a national] consensus is . . . the pattern of enacted laws.' Indeed, opposition to and condemnation of suicide — and, therefore, of assisting suicide — are consistent and enduring themes of our philosophical, legal, and cultural heritages."[52]

As discussed in Chapter Three, this national consensus represents a synthesis of the Christian and Hobbesian traditions. This "Natural Rights Synthesis," originating in the Hobbesian and Christian traditions, share this linchpin of our common morality: I refer to the natural love of one's life. In the Hobbesian tradition, individuals naturally seek to preserve their own lives. Making that possible is the reason to form a society and submit to a sovereign. It is out of fear for our lives that we cede the power to make and enforce the laws that will protect our lives. In the Christian tradition, as noted above, Jesus, like Aristotle, observed this natural propensity exemplified in

---

51. *Glucksberg*, 2263. At footnote 8, Chief Justice Rehnquist refers to *Rodriguez v. British Columbia*, 107 D.L.R. 4th (1993), 404, for a list of nations that have as their norm a "blanket prohibition on assisted suicide." In this same footnote, the Chief Justice refers to the history of legislation in the United States documented in Marzen, O'Dowd, Crone, and Balch, "Suicide: A Constitutional Right?" *Duquesne Law Review* 24, no. 1 (1985): Appendix, 148-242.

52. *Glucksberg*, 2263. For a history of the American philosophical, legal, and cultural heritage, the Chief Justice cites again Marzen, O'Dowd, Crone, and Balch, "Suicide: A Constitutional Right?" pp. 17-56, and also the New York State Task Force on Life and the Law, "When Death Is Sought: Assisted Suicide and Euthanasia in the Medical Context" (May, 1994): 77-82.

the relation of parents to their children: Their behavior is directed toward assuring the lives of their children, which in turn means that their own lives require care and protection essential to meeting their parental responsibilities. If individuals act on the wish that they and others exist and live, they have a reason to care about how they behave toward themselves and others, and they have a basis for knowing how to behave. If, however, individuals do not care whether they live or die, they lose that most basic reason for caring about and knowing how they should behave toward themselves and others. Immanuel Kant recognized this when he observed that

> we shrink in horror from suicide because all nature seeks its own preservation; an injured tree, a living body, an animal does so; how could a man make of his freedom, which is the acme of life and constitutes its worth, a principle for his own destruction? Nothing more terrible can be imagined; for if man were on every occasion master of his own life, he would be master of the lives of others; and being ready to sacrifice his life at any and every time rather than be captured, he could perpetrate every conceivable crime and vice.[53]

Kant states that a logical implication of a deliberate loss of caring about whether one lives or dies is acted out in those occasions when individuals kill themselves after they kill others.

Of course, we do not expect or fear that those who are dying pose such a threat to the lives of others when they seek assistance from a physician or others to end their lives. The threat is so much more subtle and mostly, though not completely, indirect. Those who argue that assisted suicide and euthanasia ought to be permitted by law and should be regarded either as morally justifiable, or a matter for individuals to decide for themselves, on whatever basis, are proposing that the loss of the love of life can and, at times, should be, a basis for knowing how to behave towards oneself and others. The publication in the State of Oregon of a case of assisted suicide records a dramatic instance of deciding what to do, based in great measure on the perception of a physician that his patient was losing her love for her life.

The physician, Dr. Kade, documenting the case I am about to discuss, is using a pseudonym at the request of his patient's family. Dr. Kade describes himself as a physician who voted twice against legislation in Oregon designed to allow PAS. But after Oregon legalized PAS, and after he had assisted one of his patients to commit suicide, he published his reflections on how he changed his thinking and why assisting her was justified.

53. Immanuel Kant, *Lectures on Ethics* (New York: Harper & Row, 1963), pp. 150-51.

To begin with, the desire of his patient to terminate her life surprised him. Though terminally ill, her life did not seem to him to be "terminal" but rather, as he observes,

> . . . in most respects quite remarkable. She was engaged to be married; she still pursued many meaningful activities; and she had a devoted and invested family. She did not seem to manifest any of the characteristics that I considered to constitute intolerable suffering. . . . She had no pain, maintained an adequate appetite, and was no longer bothered by the night sweats.[54]

So what constituted suffering in her case? Dr. Kade notes two interrelated aspects of her life:

> She was incapable of living the full and independent life that she cherished and that had defined her. As the weeks and the months passed, her spirit, that unwavering and tenacious hold on and love for life, had begun to slip away. I struggled to understand her suffering, a suffering as much of mind and soul as of body. Without the physical suffering that I, as a doctor, could more readily identify, I was unable to accept its severity.[55]

Dr. Kade viewed his patient, as he did all his other patients, as someone who had a right to make informed decisions, for whatever reasons, provided she was capable of making such decisions, and the decisions made were legal.[56] Nevertheless, he went through a period during which, as he says, "my soul nagged at me." He still believed that PAS should not be legal.[57] The reason for voting against legalizing PAS was one he continued to defend, because laws against permitting PAS protected the public from "seeking death for the wrong reasons."[58] Now he was caught between two conflicting beliefs: his belief in "patient autonomy"; and his belief in the "protection of the public," to cite the expressions he uses to describe his two beliefs.[59]

Months after he aided his patient to end her own life, he expresses confidence that "I made the right decision for her."[60] Notice the language Dr.

---

54. Walter J. Kade, "Death with Dignity: A Case Study," *Annals of Internal Medicine* 132, no. 6 (March 21, 2000): 504.

55. Kade, "Death with Dignity," p. 504.

56. Kade, "Death with Dignity," p. 504.

57. Kade, "Death with Dignity," p. 504.

58. Kade, "Death with Dignity," p. 504.

59. Kade, "Death with Dignity," p. 504.

60. Kade, "Death with Dignity," p. 506.

Kade employs. He accepts responsibility, or at least partial responsibility, for her death by saying the decision is his ("I made . . ."); it is "right"; and it is right "for her." He then gives reasons for doing what he was at first resisting, that is, rendering aid to enable someone determined to commit suicide, to do so. He begins by calling the decision that he said was "right for her," one she had the right to choose, and a decision upon which the Oregon statute allowed her to act. Another reason he offers is that he "redefined intolerable suffering." Suffering can be intolerable even when one's physical symptoms are not, for, as he concludes, "her life, as she defined it, had become futile."[61]

Without disputing that Dr. Kade was influenced by the viewpoint of his patient, and by the change in law from prohibiting to permitting PAS, there is a key ingredient that provides the moral basis for the shift in Dr. Kade's thinking from unwillingness to willingness to engage in the practice of PAS. His first description of how he perceived his patient at the time she requested PAS was that, though terminally ill, her life was meaningful in many ways.[62] But then he subsequently observed that, though her physical suffering had virtually ceased, her "love for life had begun to slip away."[63] It is at this very point that Dr. Kade begins to document his struggle with his intellectual objection to being a participant in a suicide request.

It is highly significant that Dr. Kade allowed his perception of his patient's loss of love for her life to raise doubts in his mind about what he is to regard as intolerable suffering. No less significantly, he treats the loss of love for life as a fact about his patient to be accepted rather than changed. After all, those who are contemplating suicide are experiencing a loss of love for their lives, whatever else they are experiencing. The loss of love for one's life is a signal that something is wrong with a person; they may take their own lives or be indifferent to, even a threat to, the lives of others. When one intervenes in a suicide, one is, among other things, trying to prevent an individual from acting upon a loss of love for their lives by evoking in them reasons they should have for loving their own lives. At the same time, it is love for life, and for the lives of every individual, that is the moral and cognitive basis for trying to prevent suicide, rather than engaging in it, whether as one who commits suicide, or assists others to do so.

The reader will recall that wishing the self and the other to exist is a moral commitment essential to moral cognition. If the loss of love for one's life is simply a fact to be accepted, there is no moral and rational basis for try-

61. Kade, "Death with Dignity," p. 506.
62. Kade, "Death with Dignity," p. 504.
63. Kade, "Death with Dignity," p. 504.

ing to change that fact. It is love for one's own life, and that of others, that elicits the perception that a suicide should be prevented, and the love of life should be restored. It is love for one's own life and that of others that helps make us cognizant of the various ways in which the love of life is exhibited as a natural, moral imperative. We procreate and nurture children, for example, and we go to great lengths to have in place all kinds of organizations and institutions that protect our lives and those we love. There is no need to elaborate that great array, such as the police, the firefighters, the military, the medical personnel and hospitals, and the restrictions and regulations governing life-threatening substances, whether in food, air, water, or medications. Our efforts to sustain all of our natural expressions of the love of life are so massive, and are also part of homicide law, precisely because we are aware of the threat to everyone of undermining the love of life in individuals and in communities more generally. Oregon's law allowed Dr. Kade no longer to work toward restoring his patient's love for her life. Once Dr. Kade could accept the loss of love for her life as the justifying basis for her action, and once he no longer acted on the wish that she live, he had no moral responsibility to prevent her from killing herself. Indeed, he now had a basis for helping her to do just that.

But something more has happened in this case. Dr. Kade and his patient have rejected a key linchpin for our common morality. Neither sees themselves as morally responsible for sustaining the common morality insofar as it depends on wishing the self and the other to exist, the very basis of friendship and the Golden Rule — and as such, bases for cognitive clarity with respect to distinguishing what is right from what is wrong. And so, this element in the moral structure of life's worth is not only an essential ingredient in guiding homicide law, but also an essential ingredient in guiding our laws generally. This is true because laws should be in accord with and reflect our common morality if they are to be just. Furthermore, laws enforce what is in accord with our common morality as we have observed homicide law certainly does.

It turns out then, that the question as to whether a society and its laws will disapprove and ban assisted suicide is a question about whether the common morality will be sustained, or at least not seriously eroded. Dr. Kade and his patient illustrate that for them the consideration of how their actions affect our common morality did not arise, although Dr. Kade had some concerns for some morally wrong actions that would follow from legalizing PAS, namely that some would seek suicide for the wrong reasons. He was not aware that he and his patient had approved suicide for (as I have argued) a wrong reason: namely, an individual's loss of love for life. The urgency then of working to strengthen and sustain our natural, common morality is not only a matter of providing a basis for just laws, but also a basis for guiding and shaping individual consciences to act in accord with those natural dispositions, those proclivities and inhibitions that underlie and sustain our common morality. Oregon's laws now no longer completely support and strengthen the inhibition against killing one's self and assisting others to do so. Dr. Kade provides us with an early, documented instance of how Oregon's legal permission to assist in a suicide can influence and change an individual's moral deliberation and actions.

Christian Responsibility for Our Common Morality

Any deterioration of our common morality, as understood and practiced, should be of deep concern to Christians. Christians, after all, continue to profess their love for their neighbors. That has always included a moral imperative to prevent deaths by providing neighbors the necessities of life or by preventing violence against them, be it self-inflicted or inflicted by others. The Netherlands, as depicted in Chapter Three, and Oregon, as depicted above, represent a partial shift away, in thought and in practice, from these expressions of what it means to love our neighbors as ourselves.

But the reasons to be concerned are not confined to what can be observed in the Netherlands and Oregon. Christians are not immune from the kind of thinking that informs the practices of PAS and euthanasia. For example, Karen Lebacqz, a Christian ethicist in the Protestant tradition, considers active euthanasia to be morally justifiable in some circumstances.[64] These she limits to patients who: are terminally ill; have requested the termination of their lives and are in enduring and intractable pain. To these circumstances she adds the consideration that if pain can only be relieved by being "permanently in a drugged state," individuals should, in such circumstances, have the choice as to whether to end their lives.[65] She offers an example of a woman who sleeps for more than 20 hours out of each day, and who therefore could be said to be better off dead.[66] Lebacqz expresses her own willingness to choose death as follows: "If my body were ravaged by disease, my spirit weary from intractable pain, my death inevitable, and my soul ready to face God, I would want to have something available to me to end my life."[67] Lebacqz

64. Karen Lebacqz, "Reflection," in Lammers and Verhey, eds., On Moral Medicine, pp. 666-67.
65. Lebacqz, "Reflection," p. 667.
66. Lebacqz, "Reflection," p. 667.
67. Lebacqz, "Reflection," p. 667.

stresses that her arguments on behalf of active euthanasia are purely moral. She is not prepared to propose voluntary euthanasia as a social policy, citing the risks: that the choice for euthanasia may be prompted by depression, or occur when diagnoses of terminal illness are mistaken; and that a policy of voluntary euthanasia can too easily become a policy for involuntary euthanasia.[68] But these considerations, important as they may be with regard to deciding whether euthanasia should be a social policy, do not, for Lebacqz, "undermine the central moral issue, which has to do with caring, compassion, and prevention of suffering in the face of death."[69] Clearly, then, Lebacqz has interpreted caring and compassion in such a way that loving one's neighbor as oneself can serve as a moral warrant for ending one's own life and that of others.

But the moral issue Lebacqz does not address has to do with the basis on which life is to be protected, and what inhibitions and proclivities are to be cultivated in order to sustain that basis. In her final paragraph Lebacqz declares, "I love life," but ends that paragraph by claiming that "active euthanasia can serve evil or it can serve the values of life. . . . When it serves the values of life, it can be morally justified."[70] In effect, then, as Dr. Kade discussed earlier, Lebacqz accepts the idea that there are circumstances in which that which is valuable about life is lost, and so is the love of it. Indeed, she spoke of choosing death when her "spirit" was "weary." This contrasts sharply with what Barth regards as a moral responsibility to make of our lives "the use prescribed by its nature"; to carry out this responsibility demands that "we cannot and must not seriously tire of life."[71] Barth holds individuals responsible for sustaining the will to affirm life, one's own and that of others. This is essential to maintaining proper respect for life. It is essential to maintaining what Barth describes as the "solidarity of all human life" and keeping it "indissoluble."[72] Barth retains one of the key cognitive underpinnings of our common morality, providing a clear basis for protecting human life, namely the love of one's own life and that of others. Lebacqz does not.

Earlier in this chapter, we took note of the view of Daniel Maguire who criticizes current laws for "denying a human right when they inhibit the individual's right to death by choice."[73] In this respect, as a Roman Catholic moral theologian, he is departing from the dominant outlook of his tradition.

---

68. Lebacqz, "Reflection," p. 667.
69. Lebacqz, "Reflection," p. 666.
70. Lebacqz, "Reflection," p. 667.
71. Karl Barth, *Church Dogmatics*, III/4, p. 341.
72. Karl Barth, *Church Dogmatics*, III/4, p. 341.
73. Daniel C. Maguire, *Death by Choice*, p. 132.

For Pope John Paul II, the right to life is inalienable and the love of life a continuous responsibility.[74] Maguire has abandoned both of these affirmations. Hence, like Lebacqz, Maguire does not treat the love of one's own life, and that of others, as an indispensable ingredient in what it means to love one's neighbor as oneself; nor do either of them treat the love of one's own life and that of others as an indispensable condition for moral cognition, indispensable if we are to discern what our common morality demands of us.

Maguire and Lebacqz could object to my claim that they are subverting our common morality. In Maguire's case, he does not regard euthanasia, practiced in limited and exceptional circumstances, as sufficiently threatening to the common good to warrant complete prohibition.[75] But neither Maguire nor Lebacqz provides an account of what moral responsibilities individuals have, and how continuous these should be, for sustaining the common morality and also function as a basis for our laws, generally, and homicide law in particular. Nor do they explore the moral concepts guiding the Anglo-American common law for over seven hundred years to prohibit assisted suicide and defend the prevention of suicide. As I now wish to illustrate, Christians have good reasons for contributing to the sustenance of our common morality and for expecting others to do so as well.

Romans 2:14-15 is one of the biblical passages from Christian scriptures often cited to document the existence of a natural, shared morality;

> Indeed, when Gentiles who do not have the law, do by nature things required by the law, they are a law for themselves, even though they do not have the law, since they show that the requirements of the law are written on their hearts, their consciences bearing witness, and their thoughts now accusing, now even defending them. (NIV)

In accord with what this scriptural excerpt asserts, Christians hold all human beings accountable for knowing the difference between right and wrong and for doing what is right. Exceptions to such moral accountability are reserved for those who are regarded as mentally incompetent or ill, or lacking the age or maturity to be treated as an adult. The law written on the heart to which the biblical passage cited above refers is the moral law, that is, the Ten Commandments. The prohibition against killing is at once one of the divine commandments and a moral demand, naturally knowable to all human beings. Homicide law throughout the world enforces this moral de-

---

74. John Paul II, "Euthanasia: Declaration of the Sacred Congregation for the Doctrine of the Faith."

75. Daniel C. Maguire, *Death by Choice*, pp. 117-18.

mand, prohibiting violations of it and punishing those who violate it under a wide range of circumstances.

Calvin, who was first educated in law before turning to theology, took note of the fact that laws in every nation punish murder, theft, false witness, and, in his time, adultery, moral prohibitions found in the Ten Commandments. This is to be expected, according to Calvin, because all of these laws have equity as their goal, and equity, because it is natural, is the same for all:

> It is a fact that the law of God which we call the moral law is nothing else than Testimony of natural law and of that conscience which God has engraved upon the minds of men. Consequently, the entire scheme of this equity of which we are now speaking has been prescribed in it. Hence, this equity alone must be the goal and rule and limit of all laws.[76]

Furthermore, Calvin expects all human beings to be naturally driven to make and obey the laws that limit and punish the evils enumerated above:

> since man is by nature a social animal, he tends through natural instinct to foster and preserve society. Consequently, we observe that there exist in all men's minds universal impressions of a certain civic fair dealing and order. Hence, no man is to be found who does not comprehend the principles of those laws. Hence, arises that unvarying consent of all nations and of individual mortals with regard to laws. For these seeds have, without teacher or lawgiver, been implanted in all men.[77]

As we know from our earlier discussion of Calvin's view of the image of God, he is ascribing the abilities and motivation that serve to foster and preserve society to both men and women in equal measure. This brief excerpt from Calvin illustrates that there is in the Christian tradition an explicit acceptance of a natural morality that guides the aims and content of laws, and that serves to shape and sustain human communities and their governance. These natural moral responsibilities are at once requisites of community and divine commands. All human beings have the knowledge, and the natural proclivities and inhibitions necessary, to be held accountable for meeting these responsibilities. And, what is more, to meet these responsibilities is to love one's neighbor. That means, of course, that being inhibited about killing one's neighbor, and nurturing and protecting life, are all expressions of love for one's neighbor. In this respect, Christian morality and our common morality do not differ. And, as I argued in Chapter Three, the moral structure of

76. Calvin, *Institutes of the Christian Religion*, IV, XX, 16.
77. Calvin, *Institutes of the Christian Religion*, II, II, 13.

life's incalculable worth undergirding current homicide law can be defended by reference to facts and modes of reasoning accessible to human beings as such, irrespective of their religious convictions.

Since, then, what is to constitute homicide law and its moral bases involve the very requisites of our communal life; and since the abilities to discern and act upon these requisites are shared by Christians and non-Christians alike, there is no valid reason to exclude Christian reflection on what policies enhance or threaten the natural proclivities and inhibitions that make it possible to act in accord with these requisites of community. The obligation to foster and preserve our larger communities is a shared, human responsibility. Loving one's neighbor as oneself is not solely a personal or private matter for Christians or non-Christians. Laws and policies that reduce those inhibitions and proclivities that help protect human life will result in the loss of human life. One does not need a Christian doctrine of human sinfulness to know that laws and policies are essential to curb human tendencies toward violence and unjustified killing. Christians and non-Christians have a shared moral responsibility for the laws and policies that are essential for protecting human life. Carrying out this responsibility will depend on a mutual reliance on what we as human beings can naturally know about right and wrong, and about the facts relevant to the laws and policies we have enacted and seek to enact. There are shared responsibilities also to teach our common morality and to foster moral development. This whole approach that I am taking at this point is currently being questioned in the philosophical and theological literature, and has been historically. I deal with those challenges extensively in another work of mine.[78]

Alleviating Suffering: A Shared Responsibility

Advocates of PAS and euthanasia express a strong desire to relieve suffering, even avoid and eliminate it. But no one should doubt that Christians have an equally strong desire to relieve suffering, regardless of their views regarding PAS and euthanasia. On the whole, however, the Christian tradition historically and presently favors relief of suffering without resort to PAS and euthanasia.

Advocates of PAS and euthanasia, as we have observed in Chapter One, view suffering under certain circumstances as completely meaningless. That the Christian tradition has by and large urged individuals to find meaning in

---

78. Arthur J. Dyck, *Rethinking Rights and Responsibilities: The Moral Bonds of Community* (Cleveland: Pilgrim Press, 1994). A revised edition is forthcoming from Georgetown University Press.

suffering should lead no one to think that the quest for meaning, even in one's last days, is considered to be a substitute for efforts to alleviate suffering for those who are ill. On the contrary, as Nigel Cameron has observed,

> The single most significant beneficial development in medicine in our generation has been hospice care, and the rise of palliative medicine as a central specialty. It is no coincidence that this was from the start a Christian project, devised by the remarkable Dr. Cicely Saunders back in the 1960s. Because Christians can face death with a steady eye we are not like those without hope. We can see beyond the grave, though the grave can have a place on our horizon.[79]

And, as we noted in Chapter One, there is considerable evidence that hospice care deals so effectively with pain and suffering that few of their patients ask about PAS and euthanasia, and they generally do not persist in the desire to end their lives in either of these ways.

Beyond the increasingly effective pain relief that hospice has pioneered, there is an important further dimension to hospice care that stems from its Christian roots. The alleviation of the kind of suffering that leads dying patients to express a desire to have their deaths deliberately hastened requires a good deal more of caregivers than relief of pain. A recent study of terminally ill cancer patients, all of whom were receiving what the authors describe as "aggressive, inpatient palliative care," found "substantial rates of clinical depression (17%) and desire for hastened death (17%).[80] But the authors discovered no significant association between desire for hastened death and either the presence of pain or pain intensity."[81] Although the authors recognized that this finding might reflect the quality of the pain management practiced in the study institution, they also viewed this result as a confirmation of "previous research that found little or no relationship between pain and desire for hastened death or interest in assisted suicide."[82] If patients were depressed,

---

79. Nigel M. de S. Cameron, "A Theological Mandate for Medicine," in John F. Kilner, Robert D. Orr, and Judith A. Shelly, eds., *The Changing Face of Health Care: A Christian Appraisal of Managed Care, Resource Allocation, and Patient-Caregiver Relationships* (Grand Rapids: Eerdmans, 1998), p. 44.

80. William Breitbart et al., "Depression, Hopelessness, and Desire for Hastened Death in Terminally Ill Patients with Cancer," *Journal of the American Medical Association* 284, no. 22 (December 13, 2000): 2910.

81. Breitbart et al., "Depression, Hopelessness, and Desire for Hastened Death," p. 2910.

82. Breitbart et al., "Depression, Hopelessness, and Desire for Hastened Death," p. 2910.

they were four times as likely to wish for hastened death as patients who were not depressed. The authors report another significant reason for seeking a hastened death, namely, hopelessness. They characterized hopelessness as "a pessimistic cognitive style rather than an assessment of one's poor progress."[83] Taking hopelessness as defined into account, the authors reported the following results:

> We found that both depression and hopelessness provided independent contributions to predicting desire for hastening death. Among patients who were neither depressed nor hopeless, none had high desire for hastened death, whereas approximately one fourth of the patients with either one of these factors had high desire for hastened death, and nearly two thirds of patients with both depression and hopelessness had high desire for hastened death.[84]

Given the data reported in this study of dying cancer patients, and given that hospice patients very seldom persist in a desire to hasten death, or in requesting PAS or euthanasia, one can confidently assert that hospice caregivers not only manage pain very well, but also greatly alleviate suffering due to depression and hopelessness. Treating these experiences of suffering is very much an explicit concern for Christian caregivers, and hospice has reincorporated this concern into its caregiving model. Indeed, Edmund Pellegrino, himself a Christian physician, notes that the Christian tradition does not bind "patients or physicians to pursue futile and excessively burdensome treatment," but it does require "care, pain relief, and addressing suffering."[85] Pellegrino very pointedly stresses that

> suffering has a variety of causes other than pain, e.g., feelings of guilt at being a burden to others, mental depression, alienation from the world of the healthy, fear of the process of dying, spiritual confusion, the dissolution of life plans, as well as the attitudes of care-givers, friends, or family whose fear and distaste for the sight of suffering will be perceived by the suffering person. These perceptions add to the desire to be rid even of life, or to escape.[86]

83. Breitbart et al., "Depression, Hopelessness, and Desire for Hastened Death," p. 2910.

84. Breitbart et al., "Depression, Hopelessness, and Desire for Hastened Death," p. 2910.

85. Edmund D. Pellegrino, "Euthanasia and Assisted Suicide," in John F. Kilner, Arlene B. Miller, and Edmund D. Pellegrino, eds., *Dignity and Dying: A Christian Appraisal* (Grand Rapids: Eerdmans, 1996), p. 114.

86. Pellegrino, "Euthanasia and Assisted Suicide," p. 114.

After indicating that Christians have an obligation to deal with each individual's own personally experienced causes of suffering and particular responses to what each is suffering, Pellegrino takes note of some of what adequate treatment of suffering will require: "a cooperative and supportive effort involving the patient, the family, and the care-givers as well as psychologists and pastoral counselors."[87]

Pellegrino calls attention to one aspect of suffering that should be recognized, namely "that any threatening illness, fatal or not, involves a spiritual crisis, an encounter with one's own finitude as a genuine actuality."[88] He expects Christian caregivers to be especially aware of spiritual causes of suffering and ready to ensure the availability of any pastoral counseling that would prove appropriate.

The responses to suffering Pellegrino advocates are very much in line with what hospice is designed to provide, and for both Pellegrino and the hospice movement, there are responses expected from Christians and hoped for from all caregivers. These are responses that try to prevent, remove, or change the kinds of experiences, like depression and hopelessness, that would otherwise fuel despair for one's life, or an explicit desire to end life, or have it ended. Comfort-only care of the kind we have been describing is not at all incompatible with finding meaning in the suffering induced by the knowledge that one is dying and losing one's powers to live the life one has known before becoming terminally ill. Cicely Saunders, the founder of hospice, has documented the importance of the spiritual dimension to which care for the dying should attend. In an article concerned with telling patients that they are dying, she emphasizes the need to be a very careful listener. In her concluding paragraph, she makes the following observation:

> a patient needs to handle his experiences in a way that will make them significant or at best bearable to him and it is he who should decide how he will do this. We cannot impose our own beliefs upon him but if we believe there is meaning, our silent steadiness will help him find his own way through. This is not a situation for dogmatic statements or general rules . . . the body has a wisdom of its own and will help the strong instinct to fight for life to change into an active kind of acceptance that may never be expressed in words. In this, and in many other things, we cannot hurry the dying but we must let them teach us.[89]

87. Pellegrino, "Euthanasia and Assisted Suicide," p. 115.
88. Pellegrino, "Euthanasia and Assisted Suicide," p. 115.
89. Cicely Saunders, "Telling Patients," in Stanley J. Reiser et al., eds., *Ethics in Medicine: Historical Perspectives and Contemporary Concerns* (Cambridge, Mass.: MIT Press,

Notice that, for Saunders, caregivers should expect patients to find meaning in the dying process, not as a result of imposing it, but as a result of their own quietly held belief that patients can and will find a way to live while dying. However, in this same article she has made it clear that this presupposes that pain and other sources of physical distress have been, and are being dealt with, and patients receive assurances that such care will continue.

Within the Christian tradition, some find meaning in the suffering that comes from facing one's physical deterioration and inevitable death by identifying with the death of Jesus on the cross. But this should not be interpreted as a moral imperative to forego pain relief. Pope John Paul II addresses this matter directly, well aware that such identification with Christ's suffering on the cross continues to be an ideal for Christians. Having affirmed the notion that meaning is to be found in acceptance of one's inevitable death and the dying process, he takes note of the teaching that suffering, especially in the final moments of life, shares in "the passion of Christ" and Christ's "redemptive sacrifice."[90] Having also observed that some Christians use painkillers moderately enough to accept some of the suffering that comes from this source so as to identify consciously with Christ's suffering, he emphatically opposes any imposition of this practice:

> It would be imprudent, nonetheless, to impose this heroic response as a general norm. On the contrary, in the case of many sick people, human and Christian prudence urges the use of such medications as may alleviate or eliminate suffering, even though they cause secondary effects such as lethargy and diminished awareness. In the case of persons who are unable to express themselves it may legitimately be presumed that they want to take painkillers.[91]

Furthermore, in this same declaration opposing euthanasia, Pope John Paul II strongly endorses comfort-only care, and the rejection of a type of cure that has its risks or is excessively burdensome, that is, not sufficiently beneficial to offset the heavy burdens it will inflict.

There is also within Christianity a more general expectation that life on earth entails suffering, and in special ways, for Christians. Beyond the suffer-

---

1977), p. 240. For detailed accounts of the kind of meaning a wide variety of individuals find as they are dying, see the work of two hospice nurses, Maggie Callanan and Patricia Kelley, *Final Gifts* (New York: Bantam Books, 1992).

90. Pope John Paul II, "Euthanasia: Declaration of the Sacred Congregation for the Doctrine of the Faith (May 5, 1980), in Lammers and Verhey, eds., *On Moral Medicine*, pp. 652-53.

91. Pope John Paul II, "Euthanasia," p. 653.

ing that results from persecution, a suffering that persists, for example, in China, the Sudan, and Indonesia even as I write, there is the suffering that accompanies compassion that takes the form of suffering with and taking on the burdens of others. One of the most dramatic instances in which followers of Jesus are called upon to suffer in this way occurs in the garden of Gethsemane just before Jesus is arrested and the day before he is crucified. Jesus has his disciples with him in the garden and, after asking the others to sit down, he takes three of them, Peter, James, and John, aside. As the story is recorded in the Gospel of Mark, he tells those three disciples: "My soul is overwhelmed with sorrow to the point of death. . . . Stay here and watch" (14:34, NIV). Then, going a little further into the garden,

> [Jesus] fell to the ground and prayed that if possible the hour might pass from him. "*Abba*, Father," he said, "everything is possible for you. Take this cup from me. Yet not what I will, but what you will." Then he returned to his disciples and found them sleeping. "Simon," he said to Peter, "are you asleep? Could you not keep watch for one hour? Watch and pray so that you will not fall into temptation. The spirit is willing, but the body is weak." Once more he went away and prayed the same thing. When he came back, he again found them sleeping because their eyes were heavy. They did not know what to say to him. Returning the third time, he said to them, "Are you still sleeping and resting? Enough! The hour has come, Look, the Son of Man is betrayed into the hands of sinners. Rise! Let us go! Here comes my betrayer!" (Mark 14:35-42, NIV)

I agree with John Kilner's comments on this passage when he writes:

> The suffering of Jesus portrayed here is about as intense as suffering gets. He is "overwhelmed with sorrow to the point of death." His response is to recognize suffering for the evil that it is and to voice His desire to escape it. Yet, He acknowledges a more important agenda — God's agenda — which He is committed to follow no matter how great the suffering must be endured.[92]

Kilner depicts Jesus, in these respects, as a model for how Christians should avoid any temptation to request PAS when they are enduring suffering at the end of their lives, because choosing to live is in accord with God's agenda. Without discouraging any Christian from deriving comfort from Jesus as a

---

92. John F. Kilner, "Physician Assisted Suicide: Today, Yesterday, and Tomorrow," in Timothy J. Demy and Gary P. Steward, eds., *Suicide: A Christian Response* (Grand Rapids: Kregel, 1998), p. 137.

model of one who is willing to suffer when it is essential to accomplishing God's purposes, I would like to emphasize, as I did in the previous chapters, that one can fulfill God's purposes simply by refusing to ask for PAS or euthanasia, even if what one does request is to spend one's very last days heavily sedated. This too, is a witness to the incalculable worth of life, and as Pope John Paul II indicated, no moral imperative heroically to endure severe pain should be imposed by the followers of Jesus.

But this description of the enormous suffering Jesus experienced in anticipation of the torturous death to come does contain an important moral imperative. Jesus expected his followers to be in prayer with him, and be a companion to him while he was suffering. And he sought of his followers companionship. In short, followers of Jesus owe compassion to those who suffer. What happened in the garden of Gethsemane contains a very urgent message for all those who are attending the sick and the dying: Do not abandon the suffering; pray with them and for them; do not shun the suffering any of us feel when we are present to those who are physically diminished and suffering in any way. Suffering in this manner is not an evil to be avoided. Rather, it is what inevitably will occur in a world in which physical deterioration, dying, and death are a reality. Everyone, Christians and all others, have a moral responsibility to practice the kind of compassion that will cause suffering to anyone who provides care for those who are suffering. Indeed, as human beings we will suffer some or at least be saddened even by thinking about or praying for people whose suffering is such that we would rather not think about it at all.

I mentioned above that such compassion is a moral imperative for all caregivers, and all those on whom a suffering person may need to rely as a source of comfort, especially the comfort of companionship and empathy. As we have indicated previously, what is currently happening in the Netherlands illustrates the sheer moral necessity for caregivers and family members to accept responsibility for suffering with, and otherwise comforting, those who are severely ill or dying. I refer to the practice of administering euthanasia involuntarily, that is, without the consent of competent patients because, as the physicians reported, the family could not take it anymore.

One should add that the physicians administering euthanasia apparently could not take it anymore either. Both the physician and family member were unwilling to be a source of that precious comfort that comes from a compassionate companion who can, as Cicely Saunders observed, steadily affirm the possibility of finding meaning for one's life even while dying. Unless there are those who are willing to suffer with someone facing death, it will be extremely difficult for that individual to sustain a lonely quest for meaning that will divert depression, hopelessness, and the guilt of being a burden to others. In a sense, without others as a companion in suffering, a dying person is forced to be heroic, or sorely tempted to find a means to hasten death. Comfort-only care requires comforters. Pain by itself is not the major source of suffering, though if unattended, it can be. But the spiritual crisis that accompanies life-threatening and terminal illness will not be overcome by pain relief alone. This crisis must forthrightly be addressed if those who are ill are to be comforted.

Owsei Temkin, a highly regarded historian, provides us with an extensive study of Hippocratic medicine and the ways in which it was embraced by both pagans and Christians in the first six centuries. One of the conclusions for which he finds ample evidence is that: "concern for the sick and for helpless strangers was expected of doctors, and that some doctors made it their compassionate concern. Christianity was to make this expectation an obligation."[93] The Hippocratic Oath forbade physicians to practice euthanasia or assist in a suicide. From the time Christians embraced the Hippocratic Oath, physicians, whether Christians or not, generally have not regarded assisting in suicide or administering euthanasia as expressions of compassion. Rather, compassionate care can be best described as providing a "suffering presence," the very apt expression Stanley Hauerwas uses to capture the essence of the art of medicine. As Hauerwas has so rightly observed, medicine is

> a profession determined by the moral commitment to care for the ill. . . . However, . . . the ability to sustain such care in the face of suffering and death is no easy enterprise, for the constant temptation is to try to eliminate suffering through the agency of medicine rather than let medicine be the way we care for each other in our suffering.[94]

This commitment to be a dependable, compassionate presence to those who are suffering is, I have argued, a moral responsibility that Christian caregivers and family members share with the whole human community. As I noted earlier, when caregivers and family members are unwilling to tolerate or suffer with the suffering of their patients and loved ones, they are tempted to eliminate suffering by means of PAS and euthanasia rather than alleviate suffering by their comforting, empathetic presence, and by any of the technical interventions that suppress physical causes of distress. Hauerwas is doubtful that natural sympathy will suffice to sustain these practices essential to

93. Owsei Temkin, *Hippocrates in a World of Pagans and Christians* (Baltimore: Johns Hopkins University Press, 1991).
94. Stanley Hauerwas, *Suffering Presence*, pp. 16-17.

comforting the afflicted without being instructed and maintained by participation in the Christian community. But those who profess to be Christians and who participate in worship and church life share with all human beings the tendency to avoid the suffering that comes from being present to, and caring for, severely ill and dying individuals. Sometimes Christians even neglect those who have good reason to expect their love and forbearance. Nor are professing Christians immune from the kind of thinking that has come to link compassion with ending the life of one whose suffering is thought to have no more meaning, or whose life is thought to be such that the efforts to alleviate suffering are no longer worth the time and trouble. In any event, Christians should love their neighbors enough to respect their God-given ability to know and to do what is right while at the same time humbly acknowledging their own temptations to do what is purely self-serving and morally wrong. The struggle to nurture and protect human life from those who would, for whatever reason, destroy it, is one that will require the participation of all those who make up the various political and social entities that inhabit our present world.

Is there no unique source of comfort for Christians who suffer, whether in caring for those who suffer, or in being threatened by death or dying? There is such a source. Jesus, God in the flesh, knows what it is to suffer. Christians have a God who has been there! What is more, Jesus died and rose again. Though no human being can escape death, the destruction of the physical body, those who believe in Christ's death and resurrection live by faith in the hope of being resurrected in a new body to live eternally in God's presence. Though the hope for life after death is not uniquely Christian, being in God's presence eternally has been depicted in the Christian Bible as a complete end to all suffering as we know it:

> Now the dwelling of God is with men, and he will live with them. They will be his people and God himself will be with them and be their God. He will wipe every tear from their eyes. There will be no more death or mourning or crying or pain, for the old order of things has passed away. (Revelation 21:3-4, NIV)

Christians have every reason to live in hope, not hopelessness, to the end of their days on earth. For suffering is at most temporary and there is no divine mandate to suffer while ill or dying without seeking as patients or employing as caregivers the morally acceptable means to manage pain and reduce suffering. Anyone who reads the gospels depicting the healing ministry of Jesus will find how consistently Jesus healed both body and spirit for those who sought his aid. Furthermore, God has endowed human beings with the natural intelligence and the natural empathy to alleviate suffering due to pain, despair, and hopelessness. Life, indeed, is of incalculable worth to God, and should be to all humankind.

Index